4995

Clinics in Developmental Medicine No.127

RETT SYNDROME — CLINICAL AND BIOLOGICAL ASPECTS

Clinics in Developmental Medicine No.127

Rett Syndrome– Clinical & Biological Aspects

Edited by: BENGT HAGBERG
Department of Paediatrics
East Hospital, Göteborg

Co-edited by: MARIA ANVRET
Department of Clinical Genetics
Karolinska Hospital, Stockholm

JAN WAHLSTRÖM
Division of Clinical Genetics
East Hospital, Göteborg

1993
Mac Keith Press

Distributed by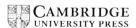

First published in this edition 1993

British Library Cataloguing-in-Publication Data:
A catalogue record for this book is available from the British Library

ISSN: 0069-4835

ISBN: 0 521 41283 8

Printed in Great Britain at The Lavenham Press Ltd., Lavenham, Suffolk
Mac Keith Press is supported by **The Spastics Society, London, England**

CONTENTS

CONTRIBUTORS

HANS-OLOF ÅKESSON, MD
Professor, Department of Psychiatry, Lillhagen Hospital, Göteborg, Sweden.

MARIA ANVRET, PhD
Associate Professor, Department of Clinical Genetics, Karolinska Hospital, Stockholm, Sweden.

GABY BADER, MD, PhD
Department of Clinical Neurophysiology, Sahlgren Hospital, Göteborg, Sweden.

JAN BJURE, MD, PhD
Associate Professor, Department of Paediatric Clinical Physiology, University of Göteborg, Sweden.

CHRISTOPHER GILLBERG, MD, PhD
Professor of Child and Adolescent Psychiatry; Head, Child Neuropsychiatry Unit, University of Göteborg, Annedal Clinics, Göteborg, Sweden.

BENGT HAGBERG, MD, PhD
Emeritus Professor of Paediatrics, Consultant Child Neurologist, Department of Paediatrics, East Hospital, Göteborg, Sweden.

INGRID HAGNE, MD, PhD
Department of Clinical Neurophysiology, Sahlgren Hospital, Göteborg, Sweden.

JAN LIDSTRÖM, MD, PhD
Consultant Orthopaedic Surgeon, Department of Orthopaedics, V. Frölunda Hospital, V. Frölunda, Sweden.

ANDERS OLDFORS, MD, PhD
Associate Professor, Department of Neuropathology, Sahlgren Hospital, Göteborg, Sweden.

ALAN K. PERCY, MD
Professor and Director, Division of Neurology, Department of Pediatrics, UAB School of Medicine, Birmingham, Alabama, USA.

RUNE SIXT, MD, PhD
Department of Paediatric Clinical Physiology, University of Göteborg, Sweden.

PATRICK SOURANDER,
MD, PhD

Emeritus Professor, Department of Neuro-pathology, Sahlgren Hospital, Göteborg, Sweden.

EIRA STOKLAND, MD

Department of Radiology, East Hospital, Göteborg, Sweden.

PAUL UVEBRANT, MD

Department of Paediatrics, East Hospital, Göteborg, Sweden.

JAN WAHLSTRÖM, MD

Associate Professor, Division of Clinical Genetics, East Hospital, Göteborg, Sweden.

INGEGERD WITT
ENGERSTRÖM, MD,
PhD

Chief Physician, Paediatric Habilitation Centre, Östersund, Sweden.

FOREWORD

It is truly said that the majority of people only see what they are looking for. Doctors and other professionals owe a great debt to Professor Bengt Hagberg, and his colleagues, for bringing to their notice the original observations of Dr Andreas Rett on the syndrome that now bears his name. There is no doubt that when Professor Hagberg gave his presentation in 1980 in Manchester, recognition dawned on the faces of several members of the audience. Now most people working in the field of mental impairment and severe disability care for one or more patients with this syndrome. It gives me particular pleasure to have been asked to write the Foreword to this book, and to have the opportunity to acknowledge all that I owe to the Swedish workers in paediatric neurology for all they have taught me over the years.

It is not surprising that the riddle of what causes this syndrome has stimulated the interest of so many people working in various disciplines. Although so far no definite biochemical or genetic cause has been found, surely there must be a defect which is operational at a critical stage of early brain development. For example, if no-one had discovered the cause of phenylketonuria someone might have been struck by the similar appearance of a group of children whose condition deteriorated rapidly in infancy, but if the child survived, led to lifelong mental and physical disability with only slight changes over the years, and have raised speculations on the nature of the missing factor causing the brain damage: as in the Rett syndrome. Among all possible aetiologies it is of interest that there could be a common factor causing intestinal and cerebral dysfunction, as there may be in muscle and brain disorders.

There is no doubt that the Swedish group of workers have unique experience of the Rett syndrome, and it is obviously important that this is shared with others involved in similar studies. The subjects covered include the clinical findings and in particular how these alter with increasing age, which is typical of the syndrome and usually establishes the diagnosis. Variations of this picture must and should be discussed, but their relationship to the classical Rett syndrome will be uncertain until a specific biochemical or molecular marker can be confirmed. Meanwhile, as with all 'clinical syndromes', it is important to establish clear-cut diagnostic criteria.

The investigation of neurological diseases has been revolutionizcd by new techniques in the past few years, which makes it of particular importance to establish what results can be expected when children with Rett syndrome are examined. It is already established that there is evidence of impaired function at a midbrain and brainstem level, which may in turn affect the frontal cortex. This would undoubtedly result in a developmental disorder from the effects of maturation on an abnormal brain.

In syndromes of this kind the statement 'There is no treatment' is unacceptable: no *specific* treatment maybe, but there is much that can be done to help the patient and the family. Also, trials of drugs, on a speculative basis, are certainly justifiable if well controlled. In fact, the Rett syndrome is an excellent model for many such neurological diseases of this kind, and for what should be done to increase the knowledge of all aspects from the development of scoliosis to the relief of symptoms.

It can be stated with confidence that this book will increase the enthusiasm of researchers, both clinicians and basic scientists, and stimulate them to even greater efforts. The importance of this work cannot be overemphasized, as until a cause for Rett syndrome is found there can be no meaningful discussion of prevention and specific treatment.

NEIL GORDON, MD, FRCP
Formerly CONSULTANT PAEDIATRIC NEUROLOGIST
BOOTH HALL CHILDREN'S HOSPITAL
MANCHESTER

1
INTRODUCTION

Bengt Hagberg

Rett syndrome (RS) is extraordinary in many respects. Already the fact that the condition almost exclusively affects only females is peculiar. The genetic background does not make it less odd. Moreover, although RS is a neurologically progressive syndrome, it does not seem to be a traditional relentlessly progressive neurodegenerative disease. Rather it shows some sort of slight compensatory gain in certain sectors of later development and in the adult profile.

Historical notes

The peculiar onset and special clinical characteristics of RS were first described in 1966 by Andreas Rett, a paediatrician at the University of Vienna (Rett 1966*a,b*). He reported, in German, on 31 girls who had developed marked mental regression in early life, who exhibited very curious repetitive stereotypic hand wringing movements as well as other peculiar behavioural manifestations, and who at neurological examination showed hand and gait apraxia. All remained mentally retarded. In 1977 Rett wrote a chapter on the condition in a large textbook series, unfortunately under the misleading heading of hyperammonaemia. Rett's work remained largely unknown outside Austria and Germany for 17 years in spite of his obvious efforts to spread information to the paediatric world through personal contacts.

In 1978, independently from Rett, Ishikawa and collaborators from Japan described in a brief note three girls with identical symptoms and signs to those reported by Rett (Ishikawa *et al.* 1978). This communication also passed mainly unnoticed.

Meanwhile, in Sweden in November 1960 I saw a 3½-year-old girl with a puzzling and extraordinary set of manifestations and a very distinctive clinical profile. These findings were first recognized in 1982—with the discovery of Rett's original report—to be identical to those described by Rett. During the 1960s I encountered similar symptomatology in some additional girls, but could not find the clinical picture described in textbooks; I provisionally named the characteristic syndrome 'Morbus Vesslan', after the nickname of the first girl diagnosed (Anne-Marie Vesslund), case S1 in the Swedish series (Hagberg 1985, Hagberg and Witt-Engerström 1990; see Chapter 3). By 1980 I had recorded 16 such girls. Unaware of either Rett's 1966 description or the short Japanese report in 1978, I presented the clinical data of the 16 girls in June 1980 at a meeting in Manchester of the members of the Council Group of the European Federation of Child Neurology Societies. It

1

transpired that Dr Karin Dias in Lisbon had already observed four cases, all girls with RS-like phenotype, and within a few weeks Dr Jean Aicardi in Paris had collected data from 11 French cases he could immediately chase from his memory and files. Not until November 1983, however, when a pooled series of 35 girls diagnosed as 'Morbus Vesslan' in Sweden, Portugal and France was published in a well-known neurological journal (Hagberg *et al.* 1983), did the syndrome, with its correct eponym, become more widely known.

Diagnostic criteria for the syndrome were established in 1984 at the second international RS conference in Vienna (Hagberg *et al.* 1985). These later served as a basis for the further elaboration of the obligatory, supportive and exclusion criteria worked out by the Professional Advisory Board of the International Rett Syndrome Association (IRSA, a parent/professional body) and the Centers for Disease Control in the USA in a 'Diagnostic Criteria Working Group' (Trevathan and Moser 1988). The first neuropaediatric thesis on RS was presented in 1990 (Witt Engerström 1990). While only three original medical communications had been published through the 23-year period 1961–83, almost 300 appeared in the eight years 1984–91, the majority in the last three years. From having been noted in only a few centres for three decades, RS is now recognized all over the world, seen in all ethnic groups and known to appear in an ever widening pattern of clinical variability.

The Swedish series now comprises 130 patients aged from 3 to 50 years (at June 1992) and is, we believe, representative for the condition and its patterns in the various ages, stages and major subtypes. The project team has access to many original record data, some dating back to the early 1960s, and to considerable follow-up information. In addition, the RS mystery has today become a challenge for scientists in a wide scatter of specialties. The remarkable onset and peculiar clinical manifestations and profile have enticed researchers to seek a key to unlock the biological riddle and to trace the background for the characteristic set of symptoms and signs. Not least, the magnificent work of the IRSA and its dynamic president Mrs Kathy Hunter has raised worldwide awareness about RS. We therefore felt the time was right to review the current state of knowledge about RS. This book is directed to clinicians and their collaborators from various laboratory fields and thus has a mainly diagnostic and biological approach. The psychological, educational and family aspects have not been covered. For these, the reader is referred to a practical guide for parents, teachers and therapists by the Swedish author Barbro Lindberg (Lindberg 1991).

REFERENCES

Hagberg, B. (1985) 'Rett syndrome: Swedish approach to analysis of prevalence and cause.' *Brain and Development*, **7**, 277–280.
—— (1992) 'The Rett syndrome: an introductory overview 1990.' *Brain and Development*, **14** (Suppl.), S5–S8.
—— Witt-Engerström, I. (1990) 'Swedish Rett syndrome basic data register 1960–90.' *Acta Paediatrica Scandinavica*, Suppl. 369, pp. 43–54. *(Appendix.)*

—— Aicardi, J., Dias, K., Ramos, O. (1983) 'A progressive syndrome of autism, dementia, ataxia, and loss of purposeful hand use in girls: Rett's syndrome: report of 35 cases.' *Annals of Neurology*, **14**, 471–479.

—— Goutières, F., Hanefeld, F., Rett, A., Wilson, J. (1985) 'Rett syndrome: criteria for inclusion and exclusion.' *Brain and Development*, **7**, 372–373.

Ishikawa, A., Goto, T., Narasaki, M., Yokochi, K., Kitahara, H., Fukuyama, Y. (1978) 'A new syndrome (?) of progressive psychomotor deterioration with peculiar stereotyped movement and autistic tendency: a report of three cases.' *Brain and Development*, **3**, 258.

Lindberg, B. (1991) *Understanding Rett Syndrome: a Practical Guide for Parents, Teachers, and Therapists.* Toronto: Hogrefe & Huber.

Rett, A. (1966*a*) *Über ein zerebral-atrophisches Syndrom bei Hyperammonämie.* Vienna: Brüder Hollinek.

—— (1966*b*) 'Über ein eigenartiges hirnatrophisches Syndrom bei Hyperammonämie im Kindersalter.' *Wiener Medizinische Wochenschrift*, **116**, 723–726.

—— (1977) 'Cerebral atrophy associated with hyperammonaemia.' *In:* Vinken, P.J., Bruyn, G.W. (Eds) *Handbook of Clinical Neurology, Vol. 29: Metabolic and Deficiency Diseases of the Nervous System.* Amsterdam: North Holland, pp. 305–329.

Trevathan, E., Moser, H.W. (1988) 'Diagnostic criteria for Rett syndrome.' *Annals of Neurology*, **23**, 425–428.

Witt Engerström, I. (1990) 'Rett syndrome in Sweden. Neurodevelopment – Disability – Pathophysiology.' *Acta Paediatrica Scandinavica*, Suppl. 369.

2
CLINICAL CRITERIA, STAGES AND NATURAL HISTORY

Bengt Hagberg

Rett syndrome is recognized today to be more common and to have a broader variability in clinical phenotype than originally thought. Nevertheless, for accurate diagnosis we must still utilize strictly defined clusters of characteristic deviant features and profiles in infantile development and in the clinical course through ages 1 to 5 years.

The average girl with classical RS is born at term into a healthy family after an uneventful pregnancy and normal delivery. Early infantile development passes unremarkably, even if some RS girls have been characterized, retrospectively, as 'somewhat placid', 'not very forward' or 'slightly floppy' (Witt-Engerström 1987, 1990, 1992). Experienced mothers with older children often admit upon direct questioning that their affected baby was 'different' but they have difficulty in describing the deviation. Such subtle early signs were first emphasized by Nomura (Nomura *et al.* 1984, Nomura and Segawa 1990). The first deviation slowly appears during the latter half of the first year and characteristically consists of a vague and non-specific slowing of general psychomotor development. Particularly, a normal crawling ability is seldom achieved (Witt-Engerström 1987). Prolonged shuffling is common, and learning to stand and later to walk unsupported is usually delayed even among the most advanced RS girls. Some never reach that stage of gross motor development. Loss of antigravity and balancing abilities are among the earliest deviant signs. This developmental stagnation is, however, so insidious that it is neglected initially. At age 1 to 1½ years a characteristic loss of acquired fine motor, intellectual and communicative abilities occurs (Hagberg *et al.* 1983). It now becomes obvious that something is wrong with the girl but the set of symptoms is confusing. Through a period of months, weeks, sometimes only days or even hours there is a loss of interest in the surroundings, in contact with parents, in use of acquired babbles or words, and particularly in manipulative finger skill, playing and purposeful use of the hands (Hagberg and Witt-Engerström 1986, Witt Engerström 1992). Medical records, unfortunately, have rarely registered such losses. If not specifically solicited, parents seldom spontaneously offer such information to physicians. Sometimes mothers have described odd and unexpected screaming attacks, which are even more disturbing for families and which start abruptly and leave the girls inconsolable for hours. Some parents have a suspicion that their child had suddenly developed hearing loss. Hence, early referral for audiological

4

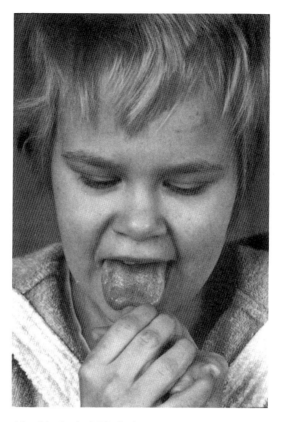

Fig. 2.1. Many young girls with classical RS display combined hand and tongue-pulling stereotypies.

examination is also quite common as the first medical activity. In the beginning of this regression, the classic stereotypic RS hand movements are usually not very marked. Initially, these are also subtle and vague in pattern, as hand-to-mouth sucking or strange tongue-grasping movements (Fig. 2.1) seem to be more common than hand-to-hand patting. Through the following year the pattern becomes more uniform and classic with more constant hand 'washing', wringing, clapping or tapping. Each girl develops her own personal and quite characteristic hand behaviour (Fig. 2.2). Most of them do it with the hands together, some have stereotypies with their hands apart, then often combined with tapping or scratching against the scalp. The regression period with the RS girl 'locked into' her closed world, autistic traits more or less apparent and with the stereotypic hand–mouth movements lasts for months or even a few years (Percy *et al.* 1990). Following this phase—usually at about age 3 to 5 years—most RS girls make some sort of 'come back' in general activity and improved eye contact and in efforts to use fragments of residual functions (Witt Engerström 1990). By this time, however, it has long been

5

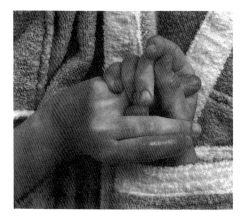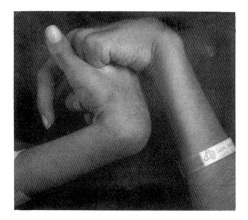

Fig. 2.2. The peculiar hand stereotypies in RS show great interindividual variations. They become more uniform and distinct with age, and are unique to each female.

recognized that the child is definitely developmentally retarded, does not adequately use her hands and is mentally deficient. It is also apparent that she has a number of odd symptoms and signs which are quite puzzling for the family, as well as for professionals as nothing described in ordinary textbooks is quite like this! Now seizures usually start too, and epilepsy is part of the picture for the majority through the following 10 to 15 years. For some it becomes a major problem. Otherwise, the preschool and school years are mainly a period of steady state. In the long run, however, there is a slow regression in gross motor abilities, the downhill course varying from girl to girl. The back deformity—a long-curved scoliosis—first becomes obvious in the majority of cases at ages 8 to 12 years (see Chapter 6). In parallel, more distinct manifestations of limb wasting and distal dystonic malpositioning take over from the previously more vague dyspraxic–ataxic and discretely paraplegic neurological picture.

It is obvious from the above that the clinical presentation of an RS girl is highly dependent on the age of the patient when seen. Some are misdiagnosed even today due to variability between cases and differences in the dominant clinical patterns depending on age and stage of the disease at the occasion of evaluation. Individual manifestations at a single examination thus easily lead to erroneous diagnostic associations when the developmental profile is not thoroughly analyzed as a whole. A regressing but mobile 1½- to 2-year-old girl, disturbed in her communication and more or less in her own world, is often mistakenly labelled as having traditional infantile autism. The mentally deficient school-age RS girl in the seemingly non-progressive middle stage of the disease with gait apraxia–ataxia is commonly misdiagnosed as having cerebral palsy of 'congenital ataxic type'. The middle-aged female, severely wasted, motor-disabled and wheelchair-dependent, usually has been diagnosed as 'mixed' or 'spastic tetraplegic cerebral palsy'.

This chapter aims to delineate: the obligatory, supportive and exclusion criteria for diagnosis of classical RS and the prevalence data related to these; the stages of the disease according to the Swedish staging system (Hagberg and Witt-Engerström 1986); and in consequence the natural RS history from infancy to middle age. In addition, the characteristic peculiar manifestations of the condition will be surveyed.

Diagnostic criteria for inclusion

While RS is easily diagnosed clinically in characteristic girls at age 5 to 10 years, it is much more difficult to be sure in other periods of life, particularly when information from records of early development is fragmentary. In late infancy and early preschool years the diagnosis often has to be tentative as the clinical features are still too vague. In adulthood, severe progressive motor disability and secondary deformities not infrequently conceal the original characteristics. Because of these difficulties, and in the absence of accurate discriminatory biological markers, diagnostic criteria for inclusion have been set up. Such criteria were first constructed in 1984 at the 2nd International RS Conference in Vienna (Hagberg *et al.* 1985). These served as a model for the elaborated battery of necessary, supportive and exclusion criteria presented in 1988 by the professional advisory board of the International Rett Syndrome Association (IRSA) and the Centers for Disease Control in the USA (Trevathan and Moser 1988). The main difference from the Vienna construction is the deletion of the criterion: female sex. An updated version of this battery is presented in Table 2.1. Definition and limitation of RS according to such strict criteria are necessarily artificial. Atypical patients, of which we now know many (see Chapter 5), are thus not categorized in this diagnostic system.

Prevalence

With the inclusion/exclusion criteria given, RS in its classical form was found to have a prevalence of 1:15,000 girls both in Scotland (Kerr and Stephenson 1986) and in Sweden (Hagberg 1985a,b). Very similar figures were reported from Portugal (Dias, personal communication). Updated information from the western region of Sweden for the birth years 1965–76 supported an even higher rate of 1:10,000 (Hagberg and Witt-Engerström 1987). When additionally traced 'formes fruste' and other odd RS variants (see Chapter 5) are added, RS as a biological concept appears to be even more frequently encountered. Thus, next to Down syndrome, RS might well be one of the most important single specific causes of severe mental impairment in females. In Sweden, RS girls are two to three times more prevalent than girls homozygous for the phenylketonuria gene.

Interestingly, RS seems to be more prevalent in certain geographical areas than in others. Thus, a peculiar accumulation of RS females has been found in part of Northern Tuscany (Zappella, personal communication). Likewise, a clustering of cases is reported in islands of western Norway (Heiberg, personal communi-

TABLE 2.1

Diagnostic criteria for classical Rett syndrome*

I. Necessary criteria
  Apparently normal pre- and perinatal period
  Apparently normal development through at least first 5–6 months of age
  Normal head circumference at birth
  Deceleration of head growth (age 3 months to 3 years)
  Loss of acquired skills (age 3 months to 3 years):
     1. Learned purposeful hand skills
     2. Acquired babble/learned words
     3. Communicative abilities
  Appearance of obvious mental deficiency
  Appearance successively of intense hand stereotypies:
     Hand wringing/squeezing
     Hand washing/patting/rubbing
     Hand mouthing/tongue pulling
  Gait abnormalities among ambulant girls:
     Gait apraxia/dyspraxia
     Jerky truncal ataxia/body dyspraxia
Diagnosis tentative until 2–5 years of age

II. Supportive criteria
  Breathing dysfunction:
     Periodic apnoea during wakefulness
     Intermittent hyperventilation
     Breath-holding spells
     Forced expulsion of air or saliva
  Bloating/marked air swallowing
  EEG abnormalities:
     Slow waking background and intermittent rhythmical slowing (3–5Hz)
     Epileptiform discharges, with or without clinical seizures
  Epilepsy—various seizure forms
  Spastic signs, later muscle wasting and/or dystonic traits
  Peripheral vasomotor disturbances
  Scoliosis of neurogenic type
  Hypotrophic small and cold feet
  Growth retardation

III. Exclusion criteria
  Organomegaly or other signs of storage disease
  Retinopathy or optic atrophy
  Microcephaly at birth
  Existence of identifiable metabolic or other heredodegenerative disorder
  Acquired neurological disorder resulting from severe infections or head trauma
  Evidence of intrauterine growth retardation
  Evidence of perinatally acquired brain damage

*Updated from the original Vienna (Hagberg *et al.* 1985) and Rett Syndrome Diagnostic Criteria Work Group (Trevathan and Moser 1988) checklists.

cation). Such concentrations of cases in a few small villages strongly support a genetic origin with a peculiar form of hidden transmission through generations. Investigations of genealogical data searching for gene sources in Sweden have been published by Åkesson *et al.* (1992).

TABLE 2.2
The four clinical stages of classic Rett syndrome

Original staging system*	Added points†
Stage I: Early onset stagnation	
Onset age: 6 months to 1.5 years	Onset from 5 months of age
Developmental progress delayed	Early postural delay
Developmental pattern still not significantly abnormal	Dissociated development
Duration: weeks to months	'Bottom-shufflers'
Stage II: rapid developmental regression	
Onset age: 1–4 years	Loss of acquired skills:
Loss of acquired skills/communication	fine finger
Mental deficiency appears	babble/words
Duration: weeks to months, possibly 1 year	active playing
	Occasionally 'in another world'
	Eye contact preserved
	Breathing problems yet modest
	Seizures only in 15%
Stage III: Pseudostationary period	
Onset: after passing stage II	'Wake up' period
Some communicative restitution	Prominent hand apraxia/dyspraxia
Apparently preserved ambulant ability	
Inapparent, slow neuromotor regression	*Stage III/IV*
Duration: years to decades	Non-ambulant patients
Stage IV: Late motor deterioration	
Onset: when stage III ambulation ceases	*Stage IV-A*: previous walkers,
Complete wheelchair dependency	now non-ambulant
Severe disability: wasting and distal distorsions	*Stage IV-B*: never ambulant
Duration: decades	

*Hagberg and Witt-Engerström (1986), adapted Hagberg (1989).
†Witt Engerström (1990).

Stages of the disease
As a framework for illustrating the strange, sequentially appearing characteristic features, we presented a four-stage model (Table 2.2) at the 1985 Workshop on Rett Syndrome in Baltimore (Hagberg and Witt-Engerström 1986, Hagberg 1989). A substaging of certain parts was introduced by Witt Engerström (1990).

Stage I
The early-onset stagnation period occurs between 6 months and 1½ years of age. The clinical profile is non-specific and additional abilities are often acquired, albeit delayed.

Stage II
This stage usually appears at around 1 to 2 years of age and is characterized by rapid and specific regression of acquired abilities, as well as personality change. In

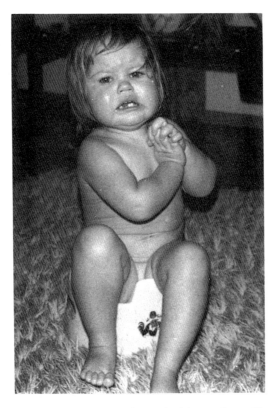

Fig. 2.3. 1¾-year-old girl with classical RS, in 'toxic–psychotic' type of stage II regression. (Reproduced by permission from Hagberg 1992.)

many patients, this stage is well-demarcated with rapidly appearing disturbances in contact and communication and loss of acquired, purposeful hand use/skill and speech. A miserable, screaming mood is common. This stage may appear in a few patients as 'encephalitic' or 'toxic' (Fig. 2.3). In contrast, sometimes it can be so protracted and silent that it is difficult, retrospectively, to delineate.

Stage III
This stage begins when the RS girl, though undoubtedly mentally deficient, nevertheless appears to 'come back' and to regain some of her original abilities and mood, and when the autistic traits become less prominent or even resolve. There may subsequently even be some further developmental progress in gross motor performance. This process of partial recovery usually occurs at 3 to 4 years of age, but can be delayed, and persists many years or even decades. It was defined as the 'pseudostationary stage' (Fig. 2.4*a*) because parents and nursing staff usually deny further regression. On thorough examination, this finding is true for communicative ability and personality but not for neuromotor functions that are very slowly

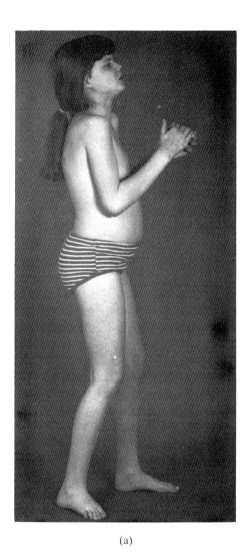
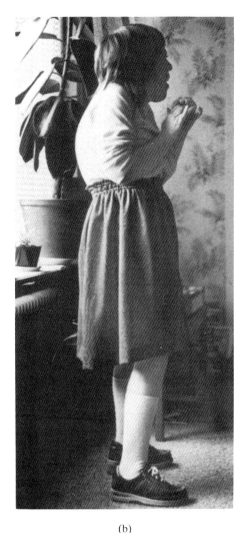

(a)   (b)

Fig. 2.4. Classical RS, stage III. *(a)* Teenage girl (S33) with hand-clapping stereotypies and air swallowing (bloating). *(b)* 35-year-old woman showing kyphotic back configuration and head retracted between shoulders.

but steadily declining in most patients; however, 15 to 20 per cent of these patients remain in ambulatory stage III well into middle age (Witt-Engerström and Hagberg 1990) (Fig. 2.4*b*).

Stage IV
This stage was originally defined as the period when neuromuscular weakness, wasting and other abnormal neurological signs finally force previously mobile RS

11

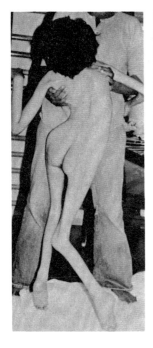
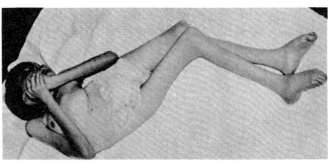

Fig. 2.5. 21-year-old woman with classical RS, severely motor disabled since infancy and never ambulant (stage IV-B). (Reproduced by permission from Hagberg and Witt-Engerström 1987.)

girls into a wheelchair-dependent life. This was often noted to occur during school age or early adolescence. However, there are also RS girls with early very severe neuromotor impairment who never learn to stand or walk. In motor abilities such girls never reach a mobile stage III. That is in contrast to their stabilization of communication skills and the reemergence of former personality and social contact after having passed the desolate stage II regression. To overcome the incompleteness of the staging system on this point, Witt Engerström (1990) introduced a complementary substaging. For RS girls who have reached the end of stage II, but already at that young age in motor impairment conform to the non-ambulatory status of stage IV, a stage III/IV is suggested. As soon as such a child starts to walk, she should be transferred to stage III. If she has not started to walk by age 10 she is considered unlikely to do so and should be moved to a definite stage IV, designated IV-B (Fig. 2.5). Stage IV-A is then reserved for deteriorating girls, previous walkers who have lost that capacity.

The adult Rett woman
Among the adult women in the Swedish RS series (see Chapter 3) there are considerable interindividual differences with respect to severity of motor dysfunction and progress of corresponding neurological signs and a surprising variation in ability at initial presentation among those who are virtually identically disabled in adulthood (Witt-Engerström and Hagberg 1990).

Our cohort in the 1990 study comprised 30 women aged 22 to 44 years (median

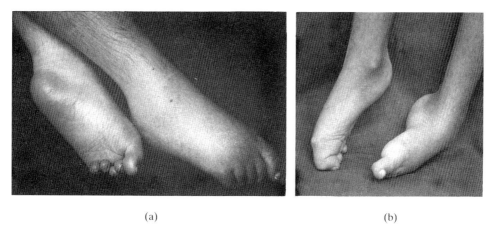

(a)   (b)

Fig. 2.6. The feet in classical RS stage IV are often characterized by special, more or less fixed postures. *(a)* Plantarflexed toes (often overlapping). *(b)* Dystonic asymmetrical postures with malpositioned cavus feet (to the right).

27 years), some of whom had been followed through decades. On the basis of acquired and sustained walking abilities three subgroups could be distinguished: (1) six women who were still walking (subgroup persisting in stage III); (2) 18 previously ambulatory girls (IV-A) now aged 22 to 42 years (median 25 years); (3) six women who had never gained walking ability (IV-B), aged 23 to 29 years (median 25.5 years). The jerky truncal tremor, characteristic of the younger children in stage III, was no longer a prominent feature in adulthood even in the patients with the best motor ability. Spastic signs, usually noted earlier in childhood, could be found in all three groups but, surprisingly, were seldom prominent. Two other main motor system impairments leading to severe disability were now dominating. One was an asymmetrical dystonic posturing with a transition to frozen rigidity in older ages; the other a lower motor neuron process with limb wasting, particularly in the distal parts. Thus dystonic limb deformity with constant plantarflexion of growth-impaired feet was a most characteristic neurological feature in those previously walking (Fig. 2.6). Among those who were never ambulant, distal limb abiotrophies with bluish-red, cold and very small feet with rough, pre-aged skin, severe progressive scoliosis of neurogenic type, as well as other lower motor neuron signs, were most prevalent. The weakness and wasting, in combination with dystonic signs which usually were asymmetrical, were considered mainly responsible for the loss of walking ability. The age of occurrence of this loss varied between 4 and 31 years. A clear tendency to early loss of ambulation was observed among those more affected by weakness and lower motor neuron signs. Those with adequate antigravity strength were less often forced into immobility until dystonic malpositions later in life made walking impossible. The importance of the extrapyramidal involvement in RS has been rightly stressed

(Al-Mateen *et al.* 1986, Fitzgerald *et al.* 1990).

In spite of the progressive neuromotor disability described, no evidence of further progression of mental deterioration could be traced either in quite mobile girls in a permanent stage III or in any adult women in a severe stage IV, independent of severity of motor impairment. Thus a severely physically disabled woman never able to walk unsupported could nevertheless have a surprisingly preserved ability for contact and communication and even an unexpected capacity to memorize. Such discrepancies in long-term disability profiles were repeatedly underlined by family members and staff in institutions. Epilepsy and breathing irregularities were also found to be less prominent and less problematic in grown-ups. Thus among our 30 women in their earlier years, seizures had been present in 28 but had then disappeared in six and were less frequent and on average more easy to control in the remaining 22. In some it had been possible to discontinue anti-epileptic drug therapy (Witt-Engerström and Hagberg 1990).

Characteristic manifestations
Stereotypic hand movements
The virtually continuous, repetitive hand automatisms during wakefulness constitute the hallmark of the condition. These movements gradually appear during the regression period (stage II) when subjects lose purposeful hand use and develop instead monotonous hand movement patterns, unique to each girl. Patterns consist of tortuous wringing, hand-washing, flapping, clapping, patting, pill-rolling, or other even more complicated, bizarre hand automatisms. In the majority, these are midline motions with the hands placed together; in others, the patting or rolling patterns occur with the hands apart. The automatisms are more intensive and complex at a young age and tend to become slower, more rigid and simplified in adulthood.

Teeth-grinding
The large majority of RS girls have teeth-grinding movements with characteristic sounds that are different from the high-pitched gnashing heard during sleep among healthy children as a constitutional anomaly. The RS bruxism is an episodic creaking sound which is similar to that of a slowly uncorked wine bottle. It appears to be produced far back in the jaw. When present, it is a helpful supporting sign, even if it is not pathognomonic.

Episodic hyperventilation and breath-holding
Peculiar and disorganized breathing irregularities are present in some form in probably all RS girls. In the most characteristic pattern, these anomalies consist of irregularly occurring episodes of intense hyperventilation, often disrupted by spells of apnoeic breath-holding lasting up to 30 or 40 seconds. These breath-holding spells have been reported to occur in nearly two-thirds of RS girls (Coleman *et al.* 1988) and can be observed independent of the hyperventilation episodes.

14

Prolonged absence of inspiratory efforts was first described by Lugaresi *et al.* (1985). In a penetrating Scottish study it was convincingly demonstrated that hyperventilation is a primary event, beginning after a sequence of normal breaths without hypoxaemia. The apnoeic pauses were usually accompanied by a Valsalva manoeuvre. During periods of hyperventilation the children seemed agitated, with increased hand movements, dilated pupils, increased heart rates, rocking body movements and increased muscle tone (Southall *et al.* 1988, Kerr *et al.* 1990, Kerr 1992). Interestingly, respiration during sleep is usually normal.

Bloating
Some RS girls (5 to 10 per cent) demonstrate such extreme air swallowing that the resulting abdominal distension may mimic an advanced stage of pregnancy. Air swallowing of a more moderate degree is common (see Fig. 2.4*a*). From a retrospective parental questionnaire study, 40 of 63 RS girls (63 per cent) were described as having abdominal swelling with hyperventilation (Coleman *et al.* 1988). Such bloating is rare indeed in other paediatric patients, and in its prominent form is almost exclusively found in RS girls.

Impaired nociception
In the study by Coleman *et al.* (1988), 80 per cent of RS girls were considered insensitive to pain. Our experience, however, is that this insensitivity is never complete or even particularly marked. It seems to be more a considerably delayed reaction to the pain stimulus, suggesting impaired rather than absent transmission. My speculation is that there may be disorganization of pain input and processing rather than a true insensitivity.

Night laughing
Sleep disturbances, more or less problematic, were reported in more than three quarters of the girls in the parental questionnaire study of Coleman *et al.* (1988). One striking finding was that 83 per cent of parents observed that their daughters (median age 4 to 5 years) awoke during the night laughing. Such curious night laughing episodes, sometimes rather prolonged, can be quite disturbing in individual patients. The episodes are not constantly present through all ages and stages but appear periodically. Often, however, they persist in some patients well into middle age or even beyond. The aberrant sleep patterns, of which the laughing episodes are a curious part, seem to reflect the basic biological abnormality in RS and have warranted special study (Piazza *et al.* 1990, 1991).

Violent screaming attacks
At least three types of abnormal screaming are found in RS girls. The first is the inconsolable crying in infancy described by some mothers as the very first indication they had that something was wrong with their baby. Certain RS girls, those who go very abruptly into a toxic or encephalitic-like stage II regression, show such

exaggerated crying in a state of extreme fear and despair (see Fig. 2.3). Secondly, some RS girls in the pseudostationary stage III have bursts of screaming during the night which seem to parallel the night-laughing episodes described above. Thirdly, some older RS girls, mainly in the upper teens or over, periodically present with worrisome violent screaming attacks nearly always first suspected to be caused by severe but undefined body pains. As a consequence, certain RS patients have been referred for 'acute abdominal pain', 'ileus state' (the bloating!), 'paroxysmal kidney stone attacks', and 'wisdom tooth ache' (one of our patients in fact had all her teeth extracted from such suspicion). This peculiar symptomatology, which may last for many hours or even days, has been recognized by parents in the IRSA as a special RS sign in puberty (Hunter 1992). My interpretation is that this phenomenon is probably centrally derived and not referrable to any peripheral organ pathology.

Deceleration of head growth
In our first international study on 35 RS patients (Hagberg *et al.* 1983) we emphasized the early marked slowing of head circumference growth, resulting within a few years in microcephaly. Thus, the head circumference in these cases had decelerated to 2 SD or more below the mean after the age of 3 years. This early head growth deceleration is one of the main diagnostic criteria, although deceleration within the normal range is also recognized as a frequent occurrence in RS. For example, a girl with a constitutionally large head at birth (familial macrocephaly) might well remain within normal limits, but show a growth deceleration which is indicative of RS. Such decelerations are easily missed, as recorded data on occipitofrontal measurements are unfortunately all too often incomplete or lacking in child health notes. In addition, 'forme fruste' cases, particularly, and also other milder variants seem to present more often with diminutive decelerations, hampering the evaluation of the brain growth stagnation which in fact has occurred.

Body growth retardation
Most RS girls are generally growth retarded, some to a marked degree (Holm 1986). The deviation usually begins in early infancy, more or less in parallel with the deceleration of skull growth. There is a disproportionate and considerable early growth arrest of the feet (Hagberg *et al.* 1983, Holm 1986). Many RS girls, even ambulating preschool children, then keep the same shoe size for years. Those with remarkably small, cold, bluish-red feet also tend to develop trophic skin and nail changes. In two of our patients remarkable one-sided improvement in circulation and foot growth was noted after operations for scoliosis in which the corresponding sympatic nerve had been divided. Similar observations have been reported by Naidu *et al.* (1987). In adulthood the very small and trophically impaired feet also develop a markedly distorted shape, sometimes with grotesque hyperflexed toe malpositions.

Jerky truncal 'ataxia'

Mainly occurring in late infancy, the peculiar truncal shaking seen in RS girls (Hagberg *et al.* 1983) is not a traditional ataxia but is better interpreted as a manifestation of a general body dyspraxia. It is a temporary phenomenon, particularly present in small RS girls just able to sit unsupported. In advanced stages of the disease, it is usually concealed by the more prominent and disabling lower motor neuron and basal ganglia abnormalities. The phenomenon is easiest to examine and best evident when the patient is held sitting as freely as possible on one's lap. The truncal shaking one feels appears to be best characterized as delayed balance compensation reactions resulting in continuously repeated body jerks. A derangement of normal positional 'input' signals may provide a plausible explanation. This incoordination differs in type from that of traditional cerebellar ataxia in progressive conditions (*e.g.* the heredoataxias). It is also different from that observed in certain static traditional encephalopathies (*e.g.* ataxic cerebral palsy).

Lower motor neuron impairment

As mentioned above, lower motor neuron involvement is, in most patients, a clinically late manifestation (stage III–IV). With increasing age and severity in stages, however, it is one of the more prominent neurological features (Hagberg and Witt-Engerström 1987). Many RS adolescents, even some with otherwise mild disease (*e.g.* one of our forme fruste patients—Hagberg and Rasmussen 1986), demonstrate early appearing distal lower motor neuron dysfunction. This is often manifested through a peroneal muscle atrophy type of foot-drop with simultaneous traits of dystonia. Sural nerve biopsy studies indicate diffuse axonal pathology (Percy *et al.* 1985, Haas and Love 1988, Jellinger *et al.* 1990). We postulated a complex lower motor neuron impairment also involving the spinal cord (Hagberg and Witt-Engerström 1986). Swedish neuropathological studies of the spinal cord (Oldfors *et al.* 1988) confirmed spinal cord and root degeneration in two adult RS women who had died in an advanced stage IV. In a series of stage IV RS girls, investigations using somatosensory and auditory evoked response methods demonstrated evidence of myelopathy (Badr *et al.* 1987, 1989*a,b*).

Scoliosis

One of the most prominent and problematic manifestations in RS is the disabling scoliosis affecting all stage IV RS girls and in most of them leading to devastating deformities. Characteristically, it is a long double-curved thoracolumbar deformity. In weak and floppy children it is often present already in the early school years. In the 15 to 20 per cent of RS girls with the best preserved gross motor function, *i.e.* those remaining in an ambulatory stage III into middle age, the back deformity is usually much more modest. Commonly, this emerges with age into a dominating high thoracic–low cervical kyphosis. The natural history of the kyphoscolioses, their neurogenic origin and aspects of treatment will be surveyed in Chapter 6.

Epilepsy
Epilepsy is met in 70 to 80 per cent of RS girls. In classic cases, seizures usually start at the end of stage II or during the first years of the pseudostationary stage III, *i.e.* somewhere between 3 to 5 years of age. An onset after age 10 is uncommon. The mean age of onset in the large USA parental survey was 3½ years (Coleman *et al.* 1988), while in the original international study (Hagberg *et al.* 1983) the median age was 4 years. There is, however, a 'seizure onset' variant type, surveyed in Chapter 5.

Fits manifest in various ways. Often a mixture of general and partial seizures is observed, usually more of the latter than the former. RS girls belonging to families with known genetic epilepsy usually have a very early onset of seizures. Often these are the initial RS manifestations and consist of atypical infantile spasms, with or without hypsarrhythmia on EEG. Many of the infantile seizure variant RS cases probably belong to this genetically loaded subtype (see Chapter 5). During school age, the epilepsy of some RS girls is refractory to drug therapy. However, these children are also prone to react adversely with side-effects on standard antiepileptic medication. Thus there seems to be some sort of constitutional sensitivity to anticonvulsant drugs which should lead to caution when designing antiepileptic regimens. In adulthood many RS patients spontaneously, sometimes surprisingly completely, stop having seizures (with problematic exceptions). Thus, withdrawal of antiepileptic drugs should always be considered in RS adults.

Normal eye findings
Well into adulthood surprisingly normal ophthalmological function persists even in the most severe stage IV RS women. Thus, in contrast to most traditional neurodegenerative diseases, RS is not associated with impairments of the retina, optic tracts, cornea or other media, or ocular motility control. However, one does see an excess of acquired cataracts, practically always explained as being secondary to self-injurious blows against the eyeballs (a not uncommon stereotypy in self-aggressive RS females). For the large majority of RS females, the eyes, and the intensive eye pointing used, remain as not only the best but often the only method for contact and communication. Their eye pointing, thus, is the way RS girls 'speak'.

Life expectancy
Some RS women live to a relatively advanced age. The oldest Scandinavian patient known is a 68-year-old Danish woman, wheelchair-bound in a rigid stage IV (Bieber Nielsen, personal communication). However, in our Swedish RS series only nine of 130 (7 per cent) have passed the age of 40. To some extent this can be explained by a persisting unawareness of RS in many centres for mentally retarded adults. Another reason may be that diagnostic efforts are hampered by fragmentary family histories and incomplete recorded data on institutionalized older people. No doubt, in addition, an excess of early sudden unexpected death occurs among RS

girls and women. Through the period 1971–91 we have noted six deaths: two in early postoperative states, two during simple upper respiratory infections, and two sudden unexplained deaths. The median age at death was 28 years (range 11 to 35). Particularly when considering orthopaedic operations, I have learned that the increased risk for a non-preventable sudden postoperative death should be discussed with the parents very thoroughly.

ACKNOWLEDGEMENTS

The studies were supported by grants from the following foundations: Vera and Hans Albrechtson, Gunnar and Märtha Bergendahl, Folke Bernardotte, Frimurare-Barnhusdirektionen, Sunnerdahl and W:6 Rett Research.

REFERENCES

Åkesson, H-O., Hagberg, B., Wahlström, J., Witt Engerström, I. (1992) 'Rett syndrome: a search for gene sources.' *American Journal of Medical Genetics*, **42**, 104–110.

Al-Mateen, M., Philippart, M., Shields, W.D. (1986) 'Rett syndrome: a commonly overlooked progressive encephalopathy in girls.' *American Journal of Diseases of Children*, **140**, 761–765.

Badr, G., Witt-Engerström, I., Hagberg, B. (1987) 'Brain stem and spinal cord impairment in Rett syndrome: somatosensory and auditory evoked responses investigations.' *Brain and Development*, **9**, 517–522.

—— —— (1989*a*) 'Neurophysiological findings in Rett syndrome. I: EMG, conduction velocity, EEG and somatosensory-evoked potential studies.' *Brain and Development*, **11**, 102–109.

—— —— —— (1989*b*) 'Neurophysiological findings in Rett syndrome. II. Visual and auditory brainstem, middle and late evoked responses.' *Brain and Development*, **11**, 110–114.

Coleman, M., Brubaker, J., Hunter, K., Smith, G. (1988) 'Rett syndrome: a survey of North American patients.' *Journal of Mental Deficiency Research*, **32**, 117–124.

Fitzgerald, P.M., Jankovic, J., Glaze, D.G., Schultz, R., Percy, A.K. (1990) 'Extrapyramidal involvement in Rett's syndrome.' *Neurology*, **40**, 293–295.

Haas, R.H., Love, S. (1988) 'Peripheral nerve findings in Rett syndrome.' *Journal of Child Neurology*, **3** (Suppl.), S25–S30.

Hagberg, B. (1985*a*) 'Rett syndrome: prevalence and impact on progressive severe mental retardation in girls.' *Acta Paediatrica Scandinavica*, **74**, 405–408.

—— (1985*b*) 'Rett syndrome: Swedish approach to analysis of prevalence and cause.' *Brain and Development*, **7**, 277–280.

—— (1989) 'Rett syndrome: clinical peculiarities, diagnostic approach and possible cause.' *Pediatric Neurology*, **5**, 75–83.

—— Rasmussen, P. (1986) '"Forme fruste" of Rett syndrome—a case report.' *American Journal of Medical Genetics*, **24** (Suppl. 1), 175–181.

—— Witt-Engerström, I. (1986) 'Rett syndrome: a suggested staging system for describing impairment profile with increasing age towards adolescence.' *American Journal of Medical Genetics*, **24** (Suppl. 1), 47–59.

—— —— (1987) 'Rett syndrome: epidemiology and nosology – progress in knowledge 1986 – a conference communication.' *Brain and Development*, **9**, 451–457.

—— Aicardi, J., Dias, K., Ramos, O. (1983) 'A progressive syndrome of autism, dementia, ataxia, and loss of purposeful hand use in girls: Rett's syndrome: report of 35 cases.' *Annals of Neurology*, **14**, 471–479.

—— Goutières, F., Hanefeld, F., Rett, A., Wilson, J. (1985) 'Rett syndrome: criteria for inclusion and exclusion.' *Brain and Development*, **7**, 372–373.

Holm, V.A. (1986) 'Physical growth and development in patients with Rett syndrome.' *American Journal of Medical Genetics*, **24** (Suppl. 1), 119–126.

Hunter, K. (1992) 'Behavior survey—older girls'. *International Rett Syndrome Association Newsletter*, (Spring), 8–9.

Jellinger, K., Grisold, W., Armstrong, D., Rett, A. (1990) 'Peripheral nerve involvement in the Rett syndrome.' *Brain and Development*, **12**, 109–114.

Kerr, A.M. (1992) 'A review of the respiratory disorder in Rett syndrome.' *Brain and Development*, **14** (Suppl.), S43–S45.

—— Stephenson, J.B.P. (1986) 'A study of the natural history of Rett syndrome in 23 girls.' *American Journal of Medical Genetics*, **24** (Suppl. 1), 77–83.

—— Southall, D., Amos, P., Cooper, R., Samuels, M., Mitchell, J., Stephenson, J. (1990) 'Correlation of electroencephalogram, respiration and movement in the Rett syndrome.' *Brain and Development*, **12**, 61–68.

Lugaresi, E., Cirignotta, F., Montagna, P. (1985) 'Abnormal breathing in Rett syndrome.' *Brain and Development*, **7**, 329–333.

Naidu, S., Chatterjee, S., Murphy, M., Uematsu, S., Phillipart, M., Moser, H. (1987) 'Rett syndrome: new observations.' *Brain and Development*, **9**, 525–528.

Nomura, Y., Segawa, M. (1990) 'Clinical features of the early stage of the Rett syndrome.' *Brain and Development*, **12**, 16–19.

Nomura, Y., Segawa, M., Hasegawa, M. (1984) 'Rett syndrome—clinical studies and pathophysiological considerations.' *Brain and Development*, **6**, 475–486.

Oldfors, A., Hagberg, B., Nordgren, H., Sourander, P., Witt-Engerström, I. (1988) 'Rett syndrome: spinal cord neuropathology.' *Pediatric Neurology*, **4**, 172–174.

Percy, A.K., Zoghbi, H., Riccardi, V.M. (1985) 'Rett syndrome: initial experience with an emerging clinical entity.' *Brain and Development*, **7**, 300–304.

—— Gillberg, C., Hagberg, B., Witt-Engerström, I. (1990) 'Rett syndrome and the autistic disorders.' *Neurologic Clinics*, **8**, 659–676.

Piazza, C.C., Fisher, W., Kiesewetter, K., Bowman, L., Moser, H. (1990) 'Aberrant sleep patterns in children with the Rett syndrome.' *Brain and Development*, **12**, 488–493.

—— —— Moser, H. (1991) 'Behavioral treatment of sleep dysfunction in patients with Rett syndrome.' *Brain and Development*, **13**, 232–237.

Southall, D.P., Kerr, A.M., Tirosh, E., Amos, P., Lang, M.H., Stephenson, J.B.P. (1988) 'Hyperventilation in the awake state: potentially treatable component of Rett syndrome.' *Archives of Disease in Childhood*, **63**, 1039–1048.

Trevathan, E., Moser, H.W. (1988) 'Diagnostic criteria for Rett syndrome.' *Annals of Neurology*, **23**, 425–428.

Witt-Engerström, I. (1987) 'Rett syndrome: a retrospective pilot study on potential early predictive symptomatology.' *Brain and Development*, **9**, 481–486.

—— (1990) 'Rett syndrome in Sweden. Neurodevelopment – Disability – Pathophysiology.' *Acta Paediatrica Scandinavica*, Suppl. 369.

—— (1992) 'Rett syndrome: the late infantile regression period—a retrospective analysis of 91 cases.' *Acta Paediatrica*, **81**, 167–172.

—— Hagberg, B. (1990) 'The Rett syndrome: gross motor disability and neural impairments in adults.' *Brain and Development*, **12**, 23–26.

3
THE SWEDISH SERIES OF FEMALES WITH RETT SYNDROME 1960–92

Bengt Hagberg and Ingegerd Witt Engerström

By May 1992 the Swedish series of listed girls and women with RS comprised 130 individuals, diagnosed through a period of three decades. The collection of cases can be separated into three main periods with different search approaches.

Period 1. Seventeen girls (S1–S17), now mainly adults, had in the 1960s and 1970s been referred from different parts of Sweden to one of us (B.H.) for diagnosis. These were included in the original French–Portuguese–Swedish study of 35 classical RS cases (Hagberg *et al.* 1983). Basic data and certain supporting signs for each of these 17 patients were also collated by Hagberg and Witt Engerström (1990, see below).

Period 2. An additional 88 patients (S18–S105) were actively searched for in all parts of the country during the years 1984–89 by an information and tracing programme, a travelling consultant programme, and a neuropaediatric diagnostic research project managed from Göteborg. This tracing and research programme with resulting data was reported in detail in the Ph.D. thesis of Witt Engerström (1990), published as a supplement to *Acta Paediatrica Scandinavica*. Basic data and supporting clinical manifestations for each of these 88 patients were recorded together with those for the 17 period 1 cases in an appendix to this supplement (Hagberg and Witt Engerström 1990).

Period 3. A third series of 25 patients (S106–S130) (Table 3.1) includes both newly diagnosed more or less classical RS and atypical RS variant females. Of the latter a number had been considered for diagnosis for several years before finally being included. Thus the period 3 series comprises: (a) nine classical or near-classical RS girls and women diagnosed in the period January 1990 to May 1992, the youngest having passed 2½ years of age; (b) seven forme fruste (FF) patients of various types; (c) nine additional female patients representing more atypical RS variants (RV) now convincingly indicated to have the syndrome. Of these 25 patients, 14 had passed the age of 20 years while seven were 5 years old or younger.

In addition to the 130 RS patients now included we also overview some recently traced girls, still under 2½ years of age and likely to be shown to have classical RS. Experience has shown us that even in classical cases the develop-

TABLE 3.1

Listed Swedish Rett syndrome girls and women 1990–92 (search period 3)

Case	Birth year	Type of RS*	Present clinical stage	Case report	Additional RS peculiarities present (four or more)**	Comments on diagnosis, deviating clinical profile
S106	1942	CR	III	—	Yes	Premature ageing, considerable ongoing gross motor regression
S107	1989	CR	III/IV	Yes[1]	†	Daughter to RS woman (S64)
S108	1987	CR	III/IV	—	†	
S109	1987	FF	III	—	†	Typical RS profile but preserved hand function—partial dyspraxia
S110	1987	CR	III	—	†	Never quite normal communication. Otherwise classical
S111	1986	RV	III	—	Yes	FF variant, indistinct stage profile
S112	1988	CR	IV-B	—	Yes	Severe floppy CR with jerky truncal tremor
S113	1963	CR	III	—	Yes	Classical manifestations at age 28 years. History data scanty. Extreme 'bloating'
S114	1989	CR	III/IV	—	†	Infantile seizure onset RS, otherwise CR, severe type
S115	1989	CR	III/IV	—	†	Severe CR, probably type IV-B, extreme floppiness, toxic stage II
S116	1944	FF	III	Yes[2]	Few only	Discrete FF case, maternal aunt to S68 (CR). Early loss of acquired skills convincing
S117	1964	RV	III	Yes[3]	Yes	Remarkable late regression variant, starting as simple mental retardation
S118	1984	RV	III	—	Yes	'Near normal' before 6 months of age. Loss of skills questionable. Phenotype now convincing
S119	1969	RV	III	—	Yes (all)	'Never quite normal'—never pincer grasp. Phenotype now convincing as FF variant
S120	1962	RV	III	Yes[3]	Yes	FF variant with only mild dyspraxia, yet now convincing after 16 years observation

22

S121	1956	RV	III→IV-A	—	FF type, late regression, partially preserved hand skills. At 30 years progressive rigidity. Sudden death 1991
S122	1943	RV	III→IV-A	—	'Late' from birth but loss of acquired hand skill and speech. 'Massive bloating' resembling pregnancy
S123	1971	RV	IV-B	—	Early infantile onset, early loss of acquired skills
S124	1969	RV	IV-A	—	Convincing RS phenotype as adult, but preserved pincer grasp, yet dyspraxia
S125	1961	CR	IV-B	—	Severely disabled classical RS with pronounced chewing/swallowing dyspraxia
S126	1959	RV	III	—	Regression first at age 4 years, preserved sudden cascades of words. Preserved pincer grasp, but dyspraxia
S127	1971	RV	III	—	FF variant with severe breathing disturbances and epilepsy
S128	1954	RV	III	—	FF variant with hand dyspraxia but intact walking/running ability
S129	1985	?RV	IV-B	Yes[3]	Congenital onset variant? Motor deterioration at age 7 years. Always hand apraxia
S130	1980	RV	III	—	Early infantile onset variant. Severe breathing abnormalities and epilepsy since age 9 months

*RS = Rett syndrome. CR = classical RS; FF = forme fruste RS; RV = Rett variant—other types.

**Additional characteristic RS peculiarities:

Breathing irregularities/episodic hyperventilation	Bruxism of RS type	Bloating/air swallowing
Nociception impaired	Episodic laughing day or night	Screaming attacks in history
RS eye-pointing behaviour	Stage III starting with 'wake up' period	Scoliosis of neurogenic RS type
Impaired feet (growth and trophic functions)	Slow but obvious late motor regression	Lower motor neuron impairment, distal lower limb atrophy

†Too young at time of study.

[1]Chapter 4; Witt Engerström and Forslund (1992).   [2]Chapter 5; Anvret et al. (1990).   [3]Chapter 5.

23

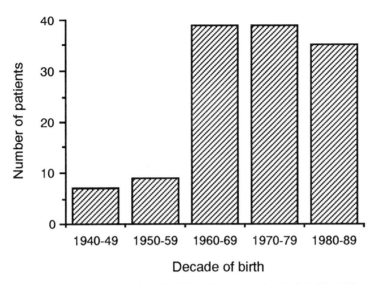

Fig. 3.1. Distribution of Swedish RS series by decade of birth (N=130).

mental and clinical profile must be followed for at least a year before a diagnosis can be made with certainty. Therefore, we have decided so far not to include girls younger than 2½ years. With such principles for inclusion and exclusion applied, RS girls from 2½ years up to women in their middle-age (the oldest aged 50) are now represented in our series. The distribution of cases by decade of birth is shown in Figure 3.1.

Within the series, 106 of the 130 patients (81.5 per cent) had classical RS (minor deviations in criteria accepted), including 11 with early seizure onset but otherwise classical in phenotype. Forme fruste phenotypes (FF variants included) were represented by 15 females (11.5 per cent); 'congenital', late regression and other more atypical variants by nine (7 per cent). Accumulation of close family cases was revealed in three families: two half-sisters (S8, S9) (Hagberg *et al.* 1983); a woman with an FF variant (S116) and her classical RS niece (S68) (Anvret *et al.* 1990); and one classical RS woman (S64) and her classical RS daughter (S107) (Witt Engerström and Forslund 1992). The accumulation of more distant family members traced seven to ten generations back was recently surveyed (Åkesson *et al.* 1992) and will be further analysed in Chapter 10.

Geographically, the Swedish RS cases are distributed over the entire country, with an overrepresentation of western Sweden where search procedures had been performed repeatedly to obtain true prevalence figures. The south-eastern parts of the country were not so well covered. Nevertheless, we believe that the series can be regarded as fairly representative for classical RS in Sweden, while FF and more atypical variants most probably are underrepresented in our clinical material (see Chapter 5).

Seven deaths have occurred in the series to date (5 per cent). Four of these deaths were caused by acute respiratory infections in women aged 17 to 30 years. The fifth was a sudden, unexpected death of a 20-year-old woman; and the other two occurred in direct relation to orthopaedic surgery. One of the latter was an 11-year-old girl in a most severely disabled stage IV-B and with a rapidly deforming scoliosis. In spite of extreme and immediate efforts in the postoperative room it was impossible to resuscitate this girl who had an instantaneous and irreversible cardiorespiratory arrest.

REFERENCES

Åkesson, H-O., Hagberg, B., Wahlström, J., Witt Engerström, I. (1992) 'Rett syndrome: a search for gene sources.' *American Journal of Medical Genetics*, **42**, 104–110.
Anvret, M., Wahlström, J., Skogsberg, P., Hagberg, B. (1990) 'Segregation analysis of the X-chromosome in a family with Rett syndrome in two generations.' *American Journal of Medical Genetics*, **37**, 31–35.
Hagberg, B., Witt Engerström, I. (1990) 'Swedish Rett syndrome basic data register 1960–90.' *Acta Paediatrica Scandinavica*, Suppl. 369, 43–54. *(Appendix.)*
—— Aicardi, J., Dias, K., Ramos, O. (1983) 'A progressive syndrome of autism, dementia, ataxia, and loss of purposeful hand use in girls: Rett's syndrome: report of 35 cases.' *Annals of Neurology*, **14**, 471–479.
Witt Engerström, I. (1990) 'Rett syndrome in Sweden. Neurodevelopment – Disability – Pathophysiology.' *Acta Paediatrica Scandinavica*, Suppl. 369.
—— Forslund, M. (1992) 'Mother and daughter with Rett syndrome.' *Developmental Medicine and Child Neurology*, **34**, 1022–1023. *(Letter.)*

EVOLUTION OF CLINICAL SIGNS

Ingegerd Witt Engerström

Introduction

A diagnosis of Rett syndrome implies a severe, combined dysfunction of motor, cognitive and communication abilities, and a growth disturbance, appearing in infancy or early childhood. Yet, the birth history of children whose later development will conform to the criteria for classical RS (see Chapter 2) is generally unrevealing (Witt Engerström 1990). The birth and neonatal period characteristically ar euncomplicated, and Apgar scores, occipitofrontal head circumference (OFC), birthweight and length are normal (Hagberg and Witt Engerström 1990*b*). In fact, signs of brain damage or congenital disorder at birth constitute exclusion criteria for classical RS (Chapter 2). Within the first two years of life, however, development is reversed; in the Swedish series, stage II signs were present in 90 per cent of girls by this age, and some even displayed characteristics of Stage III (Witt Engerström 1990). In this chapter I will trace in greater detail the evolution of early signs and the progression to classical RS.

The 981 Swedish females with classical RS described here and elsewhere (Witt Engerström 1990, 1992*a,b*) were born between 1945 and 1988. The 20 youngest, born 1980–88, were referred for suspected RS at a median age of 2 years 10 months (range 15 mths–5 yrs 11 mths) and were followed prospectively thereafter, and it is they who will be reported in more detail. Another child, born in 1989, is of special interest. The daughter of a woman with RS (S64—see Chapter 3) has been closely followed since birth, and her history to date serves as an introduction to the larger group.

Case history

At birth, S107 was considered a beautiful, well developed and lively baby with normal tone and reflexes (Witt Engerström and Forslund 1992). Her initial development was normal.

At *6 months* she was alert and responsive, and she babbled and smiled. She had good eye–hand coordination, and grasped and manipulated toys. She could turn round and sit upright with support, but would not put her feet to the ground when held to stand. No abnormal movements, reflexes or behaviours were noted, but slow response to eye contact as compared to body contact and a lack of intensity in exploring her surroundings could be seen. In addition she showed a continuing dependence on regular, frequent feeding and sleep periods. Taken together, these intuitively suggested the possibility of RS to the examiner.

From *6 months onwards* the infant's development followed a typical RS course (Witt Engerström 1992*a*). She gad a good pincer grasp and would babble single syllables. She was able to retain a crawling position when placed, but actual crawling was prevented by lack of reciprocal movements and the persisting symmetrical tonic neck reflex. In the crawling position she displayed a general flexion pattern involving fingers, toes, knees and hips. Also typically for RS, her play repertoire expanded slowly and showed little variation.

At *11 months* she sat unaided and made her first attempts to stand with support. She moved about by rolling and bottom-shuffling.

At *13 months* she seemed variably inattentive. Her development appeared increasingly fragmented and her behaviour disrupted. Fragments of normal developmental skills appeared transitorily. Subtle abnormal signs such as facial grimacing, unusual movements of the hands and tongue, inattentiveness and sudden unexpected bouts of apparent discomfort were observed.

At *15 months* her OFC measurement failed to increase normally.

At *16 months* her first signs of regression (Stage II) appeared, such as the loss of single words and the control of her left hand. She would substitute her right hand inappropriately for her left as if hemiplegic, and a dystonic element to hand movements was noted. She bit her left hand and often put the fingers in her mouth. At other times her mouth was open. Facial grimacing increased. However, her delicate ability to maintain emotional contact with people was preserved.

By *21 months* the diagnosis of RS was no longer in doubt.

At *2¾ years* she would still greet people with a smile and an appearance of interest unless suddenly struck by sleepiness or hunger. Loss of acquired skills had stopped and she was now in Stage III of RS. She babbled and appeared to understand words but would not look for hidden toys. Writhing movements of the tongue became more obvious, she had difficulty with chewing and swallowing, and she rarely closed her mouth. She frequently sucked the fingers of her left hand, and would make sudden, unexpected reaching movements with her right hand. She did not crawl and could walk only with support, preferably on tip-toe. She was hypotonic, and dystonia had appeared at her ankles. In spite of regular and skilled physiotherapy she had developed a slight scoliosis, and corrective bracing had been initiated. Growth of head and feet was subnormal. EEG showed bilateral spike-wave and polyspike-wave activity, corresponding clinically to sudden deviations of the eyes and arm movements suggestive of seizure activity.

At *3 years 5 months* breath holding and teeth grinding had appeared, and the typical jerky tremor of the trunk was present. Muscles were thin and hypotonic, and she showed pes cavus. She still moved about by bottom-shuffling.

The Swedish series

Detailed retrospective study of the 20 girls with classical RS born 1980–88 was made with the help of birth records, child health clinic check-ups and any existing paediatric records, as well as by looking at videotapes and photos and by questioning the parents.

Initial signs in infancy (stage I)

Analysis of the data showed that the disorder was first suspected at a median age of 10 months (range 5–18 mths) (Table 4.1) because of delay in gross motor milestones, usual behaviour or weight loss. However, subtle developmental variations—all within the normal range—could be traced back to the first six months of life in over half the children (13/20). The most frequently mentioned were undue placidity and an undemanding nature, suggesting a low level of social communication, plus tremulous neck movements and hypotonia (Table 4.2).

27

TABLE 4.1

Age at onset of stages I, II and III and duration of regression in 91 females born 1945–88 and in subgroup of 20 born 1980–88

	Age at onset (mths)				Duration (mths)			
	1945–88 (N=91)		1980–88 (N=20)		1945–88 (N=91)		1980–88 (N=20)	
	Median	Range	Median	Range	Median	Range	Median	Range
Stage I	11	5–24	10	5–18	7	1–17	6	2–16
Stage II	19	12–36	17	13–25	19	2–53	13	2–32
Stage III	38	18–69	32	20–51	Not analysed			

TABLE 4.2

Retrospectively obtained history of signs and symptoms presented at key ages in 20 Rett girls born 1980–88

Key findings	N	Comments
6 months		
Tremulous neck movements	4	During 1st month
Hypotonia	5	From 2nd/3rd month
Weak contact	5	Noted only retrospectively
9–10 months		
Not pulling to sit or stand	10	Equilibrium delay
Not standing with support	10	
Crawlers/deviant crawlers	5	
Bottom-shufflers	8	Locomotion changed
Rollers	5	
Immobile	2	Locomotion absent
15 months		
Hypotonia, ataxia, tremor	11	
Loss of acquired hand skill	9	
Speech delay	11	Stage II signs
Impaired contact	10	
Deceleration of OFC growth rate	8	
18 months		
Dysequilibrium, ataxia, apraxia	16	
Loss of acquired hand skill	16	
Loss of acquired speech	10	Stage II signs
Loss of interest	16	
Screaming spells	10	
24 months		
Dysequilibrium, ataxia, apraxia	18	
Loss of acquired hand skill	18	
Hand stereotypies	18	
Loss of speech	14	Stage II signs; stage III
Poor interest	18	signs emerging
Screaming spells	14	
Bruxism	5	
Breathing irregularities	5	

However, some early video recordings did show excessive, bilateral hand movements, sometimes of mirror movement type.

A characteristic developmental pattern with dissociation of motor development and delay in equilibrium control was apparent by 10 months of age. Two thirds of the girls had hypotonia and increased joint mobility in the lower limbs, so that they often lay or sat with their legs in a frog-type posture. The ability to raise the body to the upright position and to move independently was late appearing or absent, and moving about was generally executed by rolling or bottom-shuffling instead of crawling (Table 4.2). At 1 year, 11 could not take their weight on their feet. By contrast, head control was normal, and 11 could achieve a pincer grasp. Some deceleration of brain growth, as represented by falling OFC centile measurements, was already apparent in seven girls just before the age of 1 year.

There was considerable variation in the girls' achievements before stage II was reached. Best gross motor performances ranged between sitting with support only (2/20) to walking unaided though with an immature, broad-based gait (6/20). Fine motor skills such as tapping the hands against a surface (3/20), the ability to take off socks or a hat (1/20) or to finger-feed themselves (7/20) were reported. Speech was developed at most to three-word sentences (1/20), while single words were acquired by 16 girls and babbling only, by two. For assessing contact, the labels 'normal', 'weak' and 'uncuddly' were used. 13 of the girls were classified as normal or 'calm' (*i.e.* placid), five as weak, and two uncuddly. Parents told of exploratory mouthing behaviour, manipulative behaviour such as banging, throwing and waving objects, and functional abilities such as brushing hair, holding a telephone receiver to the ear, the use of a spoon for feeding and drinking unaided from a cup as the most advanced behaviour achieved. Symbolic play, though, such as feeding a doll with a spoon, brushing its hair or holding a telephone receiver to its ear, was never recorded.

Regression (stage II)
Early development was reversed at a median age of 17 months (range 13–25 months). Movement and behaviour became increasingly dyscoordinated and fragmented, and the girls commonly seemed withdrawn and frightened. Previously acquired skills of purposeful use of the hands, of speech and of sociability started to disappear; in some girls they were lost rapidly within a week, in others more gradually over several months. Parallel to disappearance of voluntary movements and abilities, appearance of involuntary movements was typical. Initially, excessive flapping, wringing and patting movements were intermingled with normal hand movements. This was followed by stereotypic movements of the hands around the mouth, abnormal tongue movements and teeth grinding. Squinting developed, and eye–hand coordination gradually disappeared. Trunk movements became jerky, and the girls looked apprehensive when any change of position was involved, such as being tilted or lifted. Loss of gross motor function was not characteristic, though it was clear that sitting, bottom-shuffling, standing or walking became more

difficult for them. Night-time wakefulness and spells of screaming and inappropriate laughter developed. Irregular breathing was noted while the children were awake, but was not present during sleep.

The established syndrome (stage III)
After a median time of 13 months (range 2–32 months) in stage II, and when the girls had reached a median age of 2½ years (range 20–51 months), a further change took place. Contrary to the clinical course in progressive encephalopathies, the children gradually began to lose their apathy and to show some semblance of reawakening sociability. However, they remained deprived of their ability for voluntary actions, *i.e.* they were apraxic/dyspraxic. In spite of these difficulties, the girls in early stage III tried alternative means of action. For example, they would look at those around them with some interest, and would indicate with their eyes objects they wanted brought to them or wanted others to look at; it is a constant finding in the Swedish RS series that this eye-pointing 'conversational' skill persists into adulthood (Witt Engerström 1990). This pseudostationary stage, in which motor ability is preserved and some communication restored, generally lasts through preschool and school years, sometimes into adulthood (Witt-Engerström and Hagberg 1990).

The characteristic features of established RS can be summarized as having the following main components, which will be examined in turn:
- a motor disorder comprising apraxia/dyspraxia, incoordination, dyskinesia, dystonia;
- a developmental deficiency including mental retardation and disturbance of perception and central processing;
- a dysfunction of communication, often comprising autism;
- seizures;
- a breathing regulation disorder during wakefulness;
- dysfunction of growth;
- dysfunction of the spinal cord/lower motor neuron;
- dysfunction of the gastrointestinal tract.

THE MOTOR DISORDER
Although no further loss of skills occurred, the girls' ability to perform voluntary movements was very limited—that is, they were apraxic/dyspraxic. Occasionally, though, in non-demanding situations when their interest was aroused, 11 of the girls would make simple reaching out, grabbing or tapping movements. However, eye-hand coordination had disappeared in 17 girls. 15 had intermittent, convergent squints; these disappeared later in most but not all. Oral motor function was disturbed, with chewing and swallowing difficulties and an inability to close the mouth during swallowing. Drooling was present in 10 girls (age 3–10 years). Truncal ataxia was present in 16; this peculiar jerky tremor was most easily recognized when the individual sat on one's knee. 12 girls were able to walk at age 3 years, and 15 at 4 years; two of these later stopped walking, at 5 and 7 years

respectively. The remaining five never walked and thus were categorized as stage III/IV (see Chapter 2). Those who did walk did so on a broad base, and often rocked from side to side to initiate the next step. Some turned in circles. Heel–toe (plantigrade) walking was not seen, but several girls were toe-walkers. Dystonia was added to earlier hypotonia, causing inversion and plantarflexion of the feet, and an increasing, tight tension of the hand-wringing stereotypies. There was grinding of the back teeth, and knee jerk reflexes were exaggerated.

Involuntary movements, particularly following emotional stimuli, are a particularly prominent feature of RS. Hand-wringing stereotypies—hand clasping, squeezing and rubbing—were much in evidence. The hands were frequently put into the mouth, usually separately, and moved round and round the tongue; as one hand came out, the other went in. When the girls held their hands together, it was difficult to separate them. These stereotypies, writhing movements of the tongue and grinding of the back teeth would be repeated endlessly. Each girl had her own pattern, disrupted only by diversion or sleep.

MENTAL RETARDATION

The girls' intellectual functioning appeared to be subject to fluctuation. On occasion they gave the impression of enjoying funny situations and jokes, at other times they appeared quite withdrawn. Responses when they occurred were delayed, but whether this was due to a defect in afferent conduction or perception, or to disturbed central processing, or to the apraxia preventing the necessary voluntary action, was uncertain. An apparently impaired perception of pain was observed in nine of the girls. Play never advanced beyond a functional level, and maturation to imaginative play was never seen (Witt Engerström 1990). In a previous study of 39 of the larger Swedish series of 91 girls and women, Lindberg (1991) found a neurodevelopmental level below 2 years regardless of age. All had been assessed as severely mentally retarded at school entrance (age 7 years).

COMMUNICATION DISORDER

During their period of regression (stage II) most of the girls with RS did conform to the DSM-III-R criteria for autism, as they lost skills in sociability, hand use and speech before the age of 3 years, and in addition acquired stereotypic hand movements and derangements of perception. In a retrospective Swedish study, 78 per cent of girls with RS had been labelled autistic before the diagnosis of RS was made (Witt-Engerström and Gillberg 1987). However, the diagnosis of autism must be questionable in stage III when apraxia and signs of returning sociability become evident.

The girls never regained their previous range of speech after regression. In 11 of them it was replaced by babbling and in addition by occasional, sudden bursts of single words. Even after several years, single words would suddenly be uttered, apparently in the right context, when the girls were highly motivated. They seemed very sensitive to body language and emotional stimuli. Understanding of words was difficult to assess because of fluctuating attention and apraxia; pictures of familiar situations appeared to be understood by most of the girls (Lindberg 1991).

SEIZURES

These were sometimes difficult to differentiate from spells of breath-holding (see below), intense hand-wringing, dystonia, inappropriate screaming or laughter and sudden absence-like freezing of activity. However, genuine seizures of mixed type were diagnosed in 11 of the 20 girls at age 3½ years, in 13 at 5 years, and in 16 by 10 years of age. Early EEG findings, which generally preceded the clinical recognition of seizures by some years, were the appearance of focal spikes in rolandic areas during sleep (Hagne *et al.* 1989). Initial focal spike activity was recorded in left centro-temporal, -parietal and -occipital leads or bilaterally with a left-sided dominance in 13 girls, of whom one was in Stage I, seven in Stage II and five were in early Stage III. One girl had a right-sided occipital focus. Later in Stage III different epileptiform patterns ensued, particularly multifocal and bilaterally synchronous spike and wave discharges, suggesting a diffuse subcortical origin.

ABNORMAL BREATHING

In early stage III, episodes of abnormal breathing were present in 13 of the 20 girls. These took the form of periods of hyperventilation and/or breath-holding during wakefulness. Most characteristic were irregular periods of intense hyperventilation interrupted by prolonged breath-holding, with air finally being expelled against a more or less closed glottis. Air swallowing during breath-holding and abdominal distension mimicking the later stages of pregnancy resulted (see Fig. 2.4*a*, p. 11). In the larger Swedish RS series of 91 girls and women with classic RS between the ages of 3 and 10 years, hyperventilation, breath-holding and abdominal distension were reported in 45 per cent, 65 per cent and 30 per cent respectively (Witt Engerström 1992*b*). There were no breathing abnormalities during sleep.

GROWTH RETARDATION

Retardation of growth first became apparent as failure of normal brain growth (as evidenced by OFC measurements) between the ages of 5 months and 4 years. 22 CT scans in 19 girls aged 13 months to 3½ years (one in Stage I, 10 in Stage II and 11 in Stage III) in the larger Swedish RS series revealed no abnormalities (Witt Engerström 1992*a*).

General growth retardation was apparent by the age of 6 years and gradually increased in degree. However, integrity of the exquisite hormonal balance necessary for normal pregnancy, and the ability to deliver a child of normal birthweight has been demonstrated by the RS mother of the infant (S107) described at the beginning of this chapter.

DYSFUNCTION OF THE SPINAL CORD/LOWER MOTOR NEURON

Distal limb atrophy, particularly peroneal muscular atrophy with pes adductus, was found in early childhood. Abiotrophic changes of the feet became apparent in stage II, and they grew so slowly that the same size of shoe could be used for years. The peripheral circulation appeared impaired early, and in addition to remaining small the feet were a reddish colour during stage II. Later they became purplish with atrophic looking skin, and were sometimes swollen. Increasing difficulty was found in keeping the feet and legs warm.

DYSFUNCTION OF THE GASTROINTESTINAL TRACT
Vomiting was common and constipation problematic in 12 girls in early stage III. Weight loss, mimicking coeliac disease, was extensive in many girls, and was already apparent by 2 to 3 years of age. This was in agreement with earlier observations (Hagberg and Witt-Engerström 1987).

Discussion
The chance of following the 'Rett daughter' (see above) from birth has emphasized an important feature of evolving RS: the combination of a fragmented and disrupted developmental progress with the appearance of abnormal signs such as intermittent hand or tongue twisting, inattentiveness, minor facial tics and evidence of sudden unexpected discomfort. I have reported similar observations in an earlier study (Witt-Engerström 1987), namely involuntary and stereotypic hand movements in parallel with decreasing voluntary hand use. Budden (1986) recorded stereotypic hand movements before loss of hand use in five of 13 girls, in parallel with loss in seven, and after loss in the remaining child. Such signs of developmental delay within specific areas of ability, followed by apraxia and extrapyramidal features, allow the following speculations. In infancy, the immature and relatively undifferentiated neuronal network (Armstrong 1992) sets limits to normal development. Nomura and Segawa (1992) suggest some 'insufficiency' obstructs the early maturation necessary to generate interaction of tone, equilibrium control, lateralization, verbal ability and symbolic thinking. Between the first and third years of life increasing cortical dysfunction and subcortical escape is reflected by fragmentation of development, withdrawal of sociability and the appearance of involuntary movements. More or less dramatically, disconnection takes over, leaving the girls apraxic and prey to the subcortical rhythms that escape cortical inhibitory control. This lack of feedback and inhibition of subcortical structures cause the vivid involuntary and stereotypic movements seen in RS. Deranged regulation of the sympathetic nervous system may play a role in the poor circulation and growth of the feet.

The early diagnosis of RS depends more on understanding the *sequence of events* than on the appearance of any one sign or symptom at a precise age. Early clinical recognition will depend on careful definition of the normal range for gross and fine motor abilities, communication, sociability and growth, as there is clearly considerable variation in the type of abnormality and the age at which it first occurs (Hagberg and Witt-Engerström 1987, Percy *et al.* 1987). Among the cases observed in Sweden, the onset of classical RS stage I varied from early infancy to 2 years of age. Among 'Rett variants' there are suspect congenital forms (see Chapter 5), and among 'forme fruste' cases, some with apparently normal development at least during the first four years of life (Hagberg and Rasmussen 1986, Hagberg and Witt-Engerström 1986).

There is now general agreement that RS is a genetically determined developmental disorder (Åkesson *et al.* 1992, Anvret and Wahlström 1992, Hagberg *et al.* 1992, Percy 1992; see Chapter 10), though it had previously been considered a progressive encephalopathy (Hagberg *et al.* 1983). Additional aetiological factors are so far unknown. There are striking similarities between RS in its early stages and infantile neuronal ceroid lipofuscinosis (Hagberg and Witt-Engerström 1990*a*). The latter, however, is a true progressive encephalopathy with severe and increasingly extensive brain atrophy (Santavuori *et al.* 1974; Santavuori 1982, 1988), and later in its clinical course the continuing deterioration will be in contrast to the pseudostationary stage III of RS. Moreover, it is an autosomal recessively inherited disorder with a 25 per cent risk of another affected child, in contrast to RS (Hagberg 1989).

Development in RS was initially thought to be normal through the first six months, or often up to age 12 or even 18 months (Hagberg *et al.* 1985). This view has now been changed in favour of a more nuanced concept emphasizing *subtle signs* emerging in the first months of life (Nomura *et al.* 1985, 1987; Kerr and Stephenson 1986; Kerr *et al.* 1987; Witt-Engerström 1987, 1990), and evolving as a result of maturational interplay with an early deranged mechanism (Kerr 1992, Nomura and Segawa 1992). The subtle signs have been described variously as a low intensity of communication and tone (Witt-Engerström 1987), autism and hypotonia (Nomura *et al.* 1985, 1987), and an excess of hand patting or waving and mental retardation (Kerr and Stephenson 1986, Kerr *et al.* 1987). Olsson and Rett (1990) in their thorough investigation found that autism was not a necessary feature, while Percy *et al.* (1988) found qualitative and quantitative differences between autism and RS. Clinically it is important to note, however, that early development for most girls with RS is within the normal range, as with S107.

The main hypotheses for *autism* are the telencephalic and the diencephalic. The telencephalic hypothesis involves anomalies in the temporal lobe, the limbic system and the cerebellum (Bauman and Kemper 1985), and holds that there is impaired cortical processing of communicative signals and impaired lateralization. The diencephalic hypothesis is based on the notion of a rostrally directed pathophysiological mechanism from the brainstem and diencephalon, assumed to be responsible for sensory modulation, perception and, consequently, motor disorders (Ornitz 1985). The abnormal interaction between the brainstem and the telencephalon might be what leads to the clinical symptoms.

The development of tone characteristically occurs during the first 18 months, in a craniocaudal direction, to allow the infant to stand and walk. Hypotonia is believed to be an expression of the suppression of 'multivariable control' of the regulation of posture, both at the level of the motor centres of the cerebral cortex (with suppression of facilitating cerebellar activity) and at the spinal level (with depression of the tonic gamma motor activity of the neuromuscular spindles) (Forssberg 1985). The development of motor function—the ability to stand up, sit down, walk, etc.—is focused on conquering the force of gravity, on *balancing* and on moving about independently. Such postural reactions are mainly a function of the basal ganglia, but early maturing spinal and interhemispheric mechanisms probably also play a role (Forssberg 1985). Dysequilibrium, in its typical form, includes 'titubation' or tremor of the trunk similar to the 'jerky truncal tremor/ataxia/apraxia' of RS. De Negri and Rolando (1990) related dysequilibrium to the archicerebellum (floccular–nodular area) connected to the vestibular structures. Cerebellar dysfunction in RS has been reported by Uvebrant *et al.* (see Chapter 8), and Oldfors *et al.* (1990) found pathology at autopsy.

In the Swedish RS girls the *play repertoire* never advanced beyond a functional level, *i.e.* they never took the decisive step from the sensorimotor to the imaginative stage of maturation. Nielsen *et al.* (1990) found the regional blood flow in prefrontal and temporoparietal association regions of the telencephalon markedly reduced, whereas the primary sensorimotor regions were relatively spared, a distribution similar to brain metabolic activity in infants of a few months of age, corresponding to prepraxis. This is consistent with the findings of Uvebrant *et al.* (Chapter 8), whose SPECT studies revealed frontal lobe, and especially left frontal lobe, hypoperfusion, as well as hypoperfusion of the midbrain/brainstem and cerebellar areas in seven RS girls aged 18 months to 4 years.

Mental development has been studied, always a difficult task when severe physical disability is present. Fontanesi and Haas (1988) reported on 18 girls with RS. They found relative preservation of gross motor and daily living skills, at the developmental level corresponding to the age of onset of the condition, while other adaptive functions were more depressed. Their results indicate that islands of motor and intellectual functions persist in RS. Lindberg (1991) emphasized the impact of apraxia, multiple dysfunction and fluctuating attention on the girls' ability to achieve their potential. She found object permanence and understanding of pictures of familiar situations. Perry *et al.* (1991) discussed the controversy over the issue of dementia. They also found social skills to be significantly correlated to age of onset. Contrary to Fontanesi and Haas they found mental age to correlate negatively to chronological age.

Apraxia may result from lesions involving subcortical structures such as the basal ganglia and thalamus, which is not surprising if one considers the close anatomical linkages between the cerebral cortex and the basal ganglia (De Renzi *et al.* 1968). Decreased cerebral blood flow in the hypothalamic area and upper brainstem in RS has been demonstrated by Uvebrant *et al.* (Chapter 8). The combination of apraxia, involuntary movements and later appearing dystonia and parkinsonian features (Fitzgerald *et al.* 1990), suggests involvement of the basal ganglia. An affected area of brain cannot play any direct role in causing positive symptoms, which are produced secondarily by the action of remaining areas of brain that have been released from the influence of the affected part. They are known as 'release phenomena', and in RS would be represented by the involuntary, extrapyramidal movements. In contrast, the negative symptoms are likely to be due directly to loss of function of the damaged part, and in RS appear as apraxia, and later as dystonia and spinal tract dysfunction. Amount and speed of movement is regulated in the basal ganglia. Lesions of the putamen or subthalamic nucleus produce an excess of spontaneous movement (hyperkinesia). Lesions of the substantia nigra or globus pallidus reduce speed of voluntary movement (bradykinesia) and produce lack of spontaneous movement (akinesia). Lesions of the caudate affect complex behaviours and cognitive functions, probably because they interrupt the processing of afferents from frontal association cortex. In adults, apraxia is particularly common in patients with left hemisphere lesions, who often have aphasia as well, and with lesions of the anterior part of the corpus callosum (Njiokitjien 1988). Both types of lesion have been interpreted as producing 'disconnection syndromes', disconnecting areas of the brain which receive the instruction to formulate the idea of movement, from the final effector areas of the motor system. Lesions of the lower parts of areas 5 and 7 in the left hemisphere can lead to pronounced bilateral apraxia of the limbs (but not face). Galaburda (1984) suggested that this may be a 'master control system', receiving inputs from all sensory modalities and projecting to frontal motor areas on both sides of the brain. All the actions with which a child is familiar are stored in the brain as 'motor concepts'. These motor concepts, or their separate components, can be lost or become inaccessible. In RS, loss of hand use is illustrated by the method commonly used by the girls to feed themselves after regression: in place of earlier finger-feeding, they now reach for the food with their mouth. In a phylogenetic perspective, this would mean regression to pre-praxis. Initially, ideomotor praxis precedes speech. In the course of phylogenesis, the manipulative functions of the mouth were taken over by the upper extremities, and there was a transition from the mouth merely making sounds to actual speech. As phylogenesis advanced, the mouth and the hands divided the tasks. The cortical fields for manual motor function and for speech are in quite close proximity and also underwent structural changes, particularly in a frontal direction, and *left–right differences* came into being. The oral area allowed manipulation to be taken over by the manual areas so that praxis of the mouth changed (became refined) in speech (Njiokitjien 1988). It is interesting to note that the first or most pronounced EEG abnormalities found in 13 out of 14 girls with RS were located to left temporo-parieto-frontal areas (Witt Engerström 1992a). The predominant early post-regression preference for use of the left hand over the right, in combination with rolandic spike activity dominating in left central leads in EEGs appearing at the time of regression with loss of speech and hand use, may reflect an underlying dysfunction/disease process which early on involves the motor cortex. Hyperexcitability of the Betz cells of the motor cortex of girls aged 5 to 9 years has also been reported (Kerr *et al.* 1990).

The nature of the *breathing irregularities* remains obscure. Kerr *et al.* (1990) found an association between episodes of respiratory dysrhythmia and exacerbation of stereotypic movements. Kerr (1992) also observed a consistent appearance of episodes of non-epileptic EEG slow activity during normal breathing, and a failure to produce a normal slow wave response to intense hyperventilation. Lugaresi and Cirignotta (1982) used the term 'respiratory apraxia' to describe a particular pattern of breathing during wakefulness, characterized by apnoeic episodes with interspersed irregular respiratory movements followed by hyperventilation in two patients. Lugaresi *et al.* (1985) suggested that the peculiar breathing disorder observed in RS reflects involvement of the behavioural control system of respiration, and that this occurs as part of the more general impairment of other basic vital functions.

The most characteristic and vivid signs of RS present early in stage III may be characterized as the *period of frenzy and frustration*, because of the huge efforts of the girls to achieve voluntary control, with the repeated failures that follow the frenetic involuntary and stereotypic movements released. With time this intensity abates and life seems to be more endurable. Seizures often decrease. Stereotypies and other involuntary movements become less interfering and voluntary hand movements more accessible in adult life. Gross motor abilities, however, decrease as a consequence of dystonia, rigidity and wasting. Scolioses and foot deformities show a progressive course, as do the derangements of peripheral circulation and growth (Witt-Engerström and Hagberg 1990).

Conclusion

The early signs of RS and their sequential occurrence can best be interpreted as a reflection of dysfunction or damage to certain neural circuits at cortical and subcortical levels at an early stage of development. This deprives the girls of necessary control mechanisms, resulting in very immature and deranged behavioural and motor patterns. Dysfunction of communication, breathing, growth, circulation and the gastrointestinal tract also result, and mental retardation and seizures appear.

ACKNOWLEDGEMENTS

This study was supported by grants from the Folke Bernardotte Foundation, the Sigurd and Else Golje Memorial Foundation, the Swedish Society for Medical Research, the Medical Research Foundations of Östersund Hospital and Umeå University, and the Marcus and Amelia Wallenberg Foundation.

REFERENCES

Åkesson, H-O., Hagberg, B., Wahlström, J., Witt Engerström, I. (1992) 'Rett syndrome: a search for gene sources.' *American Journal of Medical Genetics*, **42**, 104–108.
Anvret, M., Wahlström, J. (1992) 'Genetics of the Rett syndrome.' *Brain and Development*, **14** (Suppl.), S101–S103.

Armstrong, D. D. (1992) 'The neuropathology of the Rett syndrome.' *Brain and Development*, **14** (Suppl.), S89–S98.

Bauman, M., Kemper, T. L. (1985) 'Histoanatomic observations of the brain in early infantile autism.' *Neurology*, **35**, 866–874.

Budden, S. (1986) 'Rett syndrome: studies of 13 affected girls.' *American Journal of Medical Genetics*, **24** (Suppl. 1), 99–109.

De Negri, M., Rolando, S. (1990) 'Child ataxias: a developmental perspective.' *Brain and Development*, **12**, 195–201.

De Renzi, E., Pieczuro, A., Vignolo, L.A. (1968) 'Ideational apraxia: a quantitative study.' *Neuropsychologia*, **6**, 41–52.

Fitzgerald, P.M., Jankovic, J., Glaze, D.G., Schultz, R., Percy, A.K. (1990) 'Extrapyramidal involvement in Rett's syndrome.' *Neurology*, **40**, 293–295.

Fontanesi, J., Haas, R.H. (1988) 'Cognitive profile of Rett syndrome.' *Journal of Child Neurology*, **3** (Suppl.) S20–S24.

Forssberg, H. (1985) 'Ontogeny of human locomotor control: 1. Infant stepping, supported locomotion and transition to independent locomotion.' *Experimental Brain Research*, **57**, 480–493.

Galaburda, A.M. (1984) 'Anatomical asymmetries.' *In:* Geschwind, N., Galaburda, A.M. (Eds) *Cerebral Dominance. The Biological Foundations.* Cambridge University Press, pp. 11–25.

Hagberg, B. (1989) 'Rett syndrome: clinical peculiarities, diagnostic approach and possible cause.' *Pediatric Neurology*, **5**, 75–83.

—— Rasmussen, P. (1986) '"Forme fruste" of Rett syndrome—a case report.' *American Journal of Medical Genetics*, **24** (Suppl. 1), 175–181.

—— Witt-Engerström, I. (1986) 'Rett syndrome: a suggested staging system for describing impairment profile with increasing age towards adolescence.' *American Journal of Medical Genetics*, **24** (Suppl. 1), 47–59.

—— —— (1987) 'Rett syndrome: epidemiology and nosology—progress in knowledge 1986—a conference communication.' *Brain and Development*, **9**, 451–457.

—— —— (1990*a*) 'Early stages of Rett syndrome and infantile neuronal ceroid lipofuscinosis—a difficult differential diagnosis.' *Brain and Development*, **12**, 20–22.

—— —— (1990*b*) 'Swedish Rett syndrome basic data register 1960–90.' *Acta Paediatrica Scandinavica*, Suppl. 369, 43–54. (*Appendix.*)

—— Aicardi, J., Dias, K., Ramos, O. (1983) 'A progressive syndrome of autism, dementia, ataxia and loss of purposeful hand use in girls: Rett's syndrome—report of 35 cases.' *Annals of Neurology*, **14**, 471–479.

—— Goutières, F., Hanefeld, F., Rett, A., Wilson, J. (1985) 'Rett syndrome—criteria for inclusion and exclusion.' *Brain and Development*, **7**, 372–373.

—— Naidu, S., Percy, A.K. (1992) 'Tokyo symposium on Rett syndrome: Neurobiological approach—concluding remarks and epilogue.' *Brain and Development*, **14** (Suppl.), S151–S153.

Hagne, I., Witt-Engerström, I., Hagberg, B. (1989) 'EEG development in Rett syndrome. A study of 30 cases.' *Electroencephalography and Clinical Neurophysiology*, **72**, 1–6.

Kerr, A.M. (1992) 'A review of the respiratory disorder in the Rett syndrome.' *Brain and Development*, **14** (Suppl.), S43–S45.

—— Stephenson, J.B.P. (1986) 'A study of the natural history of Rett syndrome in 23 girls.' *American Journal of Medical Genetics*, **24** (Suppl. 1), 77–83.

—— Montague, J., Stephenson, J.B.P. (1987) 'The hands, and the mind, pre- and post-regression, in Rett syndrome.' *Brain and Development*, **9**, 487–490.

—— Southall, D., Amos, P., Cooper, R., Samuels, M., Mitchell, J., Stephenson, J. (1990) 'Correlation of the electroencephalogram, respiration and movement in the Rett syndrome.' *Brain and Development*, **12**, 61–68.

Lindberg, B. (1991) *Dealing with Rett Syndrome—a Practical Guide for Parents, Teachers and Psychologists.* Toronto: Hogrefe & Huber.

Lugaresi, E., Cirignotta, F. (1982) 'An unusual type of respiratory apraxia.' *In:* Broughton, R.J. (Ed.) *Henri Gastaut and the Marseilles School's Contribution to the Neurosciences.* Amsterdam: Elsevier, pp. 317–322.

—— —— Montagna, P. (1985) 'Abnormal breathing in the Rett syndrome.' *Brain and Development*, **7**, 329–333.

Nielsen, J.B., Friberg, L., Lou, H., Lassen, N.A., Sam, I.L.K. (1990) 'Immature pattern of brain activity in Rett syndrome.' *Archives of Neurology*, **47**, 982–986.

Njiokitjien, C. (1988) 'Developmental dyspraxia.' *In:* Njiokitjien, C. (Ed.) *Pediatric Behavioural Neurology, Vol. 1.* Amsterdam: Nedbook International, pp. 266–285.

Nomura, Y., Segawa, M. (1992) 'Motor symptoms of the Rett syndrome: abnormal muscle tone, posture, locomotion and stereotyped movement.' *Brain and Development*, **14** (Suppl.), S21–S28.

—— —— Higurashi, M. (1985) 'Rett syndrome—an early catecholamine and indolamine deficient disorder?' *Brain and Development*, **7**, 334–341.

—— Honda, K., Segawa, M. (1987) 'Pathophysiology of Rett syndrome.' *Brain and Development*, **9**, 506–513.

Olsson, B., Rett, A. (1990) 'A review of the Rett syndrome with a theory of autism.' *Brain and Development*, **12**, 11–15.

Oldfors, A., Sourander, P., Armstrong, D.L., Percy, A.K., Witt Engerström, I., Hagberg, B.A. (1990) *Pediatric Neurology*, **6**, 310–314.

Ornitz, E.M. (1985) 'Neurophysiology of infantile autism.' *Journal of the American Academy of Child Psychiatry*, **24**, 251–262.

Percy, A.K. (1992) 'The Rett syndrome: the recent advances in genetic studies in the USA.' *Brain and Development*, **14** (Suppl.), S104–S105.

—— Zoghbi, H.J., Glaze, D.G. (1987) 'Rett syndrome: discrimination of typical and variant forms.' *Brain and Development*, **9**, 458–461.

—— —— Lewis, K.R., Jankovic, J. (1988) 'Rett syndrome: qualitative and quantitative differentiation from autism.' *Journal of Child Neurology*, **3** (Suppl.), S65–S67.

Perry, A., Sarlo-McGarvey, N., Haddad, C. (1991) 'Cognitive and adaptive functioning in 28 girls with Rett syndrome.' *Journal of Autism and Developmental Disorders*, **21**, 551–556.

Santavuori, P. (1982) 'Clinical findings in 69 patients with infantile type of neuronal ceroid lipofuscinosis.' *In:* Armstrong, D., Koppang, N., Rider, J.A. (Eds) *Ceroid Lipofuscinosis (Batten's Disease).* New York: Elsevier, pp. 23–33.

—— (1988) 'Neuronal ceroid-lipofuscinosis in childhood.' *Brain and Development*, **10**, 80–83.

—— Haltia, M., Rapola, J. (1974) 'Infantile type of so-called neuronal ceroid-lipofuscinosis.' *Developmental Medicine and Child Neurology*, **16**, 644–653.

Witt-Engerström, I. (1987) 'Rett syndrome: a retrospective pilot study on potential early predictive symptomatology,' *Brain and Development*, **9**, 481–486.

—— (1990) 'Rett syndrome in Sweden. Neurodevelopment – Disability – Pathophysiology.' *Acta Paediatrica Scandinavica*, Suppl. 369.

—— (1992*a*) 'Age-related occurrence of signs and symptoms in the Rett syndrome.' *Brain and Development*, **14** (Suppl.), S11–S20.

—— (1992*b*) 'Rett syndrome: the late infantile regression period—a retrospective analysis of 91 cases.' *Acta Paediatrica*, **81**, 167–172.

—— Forslund, M. (1992) 'Mother and daughter with Rett syndrome.' *Developmental Medicine and Child Neurology*, **34**, 1022–1023. (*Letter.*)

—— Gillberg, C. (1987) 'Rett syndrome in Sweden.' *Journal of Autism and Developmental Disorders*, **17**, 149–150.

—— Hagberg, B. (1990) 'Rett syndrome: gross motor disability and neural impairment in adults.' *Brain and Development*, **12**, 23–26.

5
RETT VARIANTS – RETTOID PHENOTYPES

Bengt Hagberg and Christopher Gillberg

Introduction

The recent awareness of Rett syndrome has added an important and not uncommon category to the long list of conditions which need to be considered in the differential diagnosis of developmental disorders. This is more difficult in the very young age group. An increasing number of young children are referred to developmental medicine and child psychiatry clinics with the tentative diagnosis of 'RS?' or 'RS variant?' or with the question, 'Can RS be excluded?' In services for adolescents and adults with mental retardation there is a growing interest in RS, which is now acknowledged as a diagnostic option in previously un- or mis-diagnosed cases. This means that we are faced with an increasing number of patients who present with a nucleus of the RS phenotype, but who show considerable variation in type and age of onset, severity of impairments and profile of clinical course. In itself, this is as it should be, given that the current diagnostic criteria for RS (Hagberg *et al.* 1985, Trevathan *et al.* 1988) are strictly inclusive and, by necessity, artificially restrictive. As long as there is a lack of specific biological markers for RS there is no certain way of determining which of the RS variants or 'borderline' cases should be accepted as 'true' RS cases. In the search for such markers it is essential to keep the diagnostic criteria narrow and even 'overly' restrictive. Nevertheless, there is growing recognition that RS may not be as clinically distinct as suggested by these criteria. The different types of 'Rettoid' variants that we have come across in the literature or encountered ourselves are outlined in Table 5.1. Based on our clinical experience, Figure 5.1 illustrates their relative contribution to the 'RS spectrum'.

The question arises in clinical practice, which of these variants should be taken to represent *variants of true RS*, which to represent *possible (borderline) RS* and which are *probably not RS but show phenotypic manifestations suggestive of RS*?

In this chapter we survey the literature and our own clinical experience, illustrating the main pattern of types by case descriptions.

Forme fruste RS

The term 'forme fruste RS' was coined for variants with a milder, incomplete and protracted clinical course (Hagberg and Rasmussen 1986, Hagberg and Witt-Engerström 1986). In our experience, this is the most common variant of 'non-classical' RS, constituting 10 to 15 per cent of cases in our Swedish RS series depending on level of lowest age for inclusion (see Chapter 3).

TABLE 5.1

Types of Rett syndrome variants reported in the literature

Rett syndrome variant	References
Forme fruste	Hagberg and Rasmussen (1986)
	Hagberg and Witt-Engerström (1986)
	Suzuki et al. (1986)
	Rossiter and Callaghan (1987)
	Anvret et al. (1990)
	Zappella (1992)
Infantile seizure onset variant	Hanefeld (1985)
	Goutières and Aicardi (1986)
	Hagberg and Witt-Engerström (1986, 1987)
	Maia et al. (1986)
	Gillberg (1989)
Congenital RS	Nomura et al. (1985)
	Rolando (1985)
	Al-Mateen et al. (1986)
	Hagberg and Witt-Engerström (1986)
	Goutières and Aicardi (1987)
	Oguro et al. (1990)
	Lin et al. (1991)
Late childhood regression variant	Gillberg (1989)
Familial atypical variant	Coleman et al. (1987)
	Gillberg et al. (1990)
Male 'Rettoid' cases	Gillberg (1989)
	Coleman (1990)
	Eeg-Olofsson et al. (1990)
	Philippart (1990)
	Topçu et al. (1991)

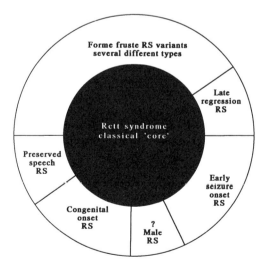

Fig. 5.1. Spectrum of 'Rettoid' phenotypes, including classical core group and wide range of variants, showing their distribution according to our clinical experience.

41

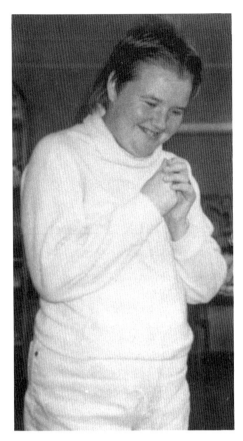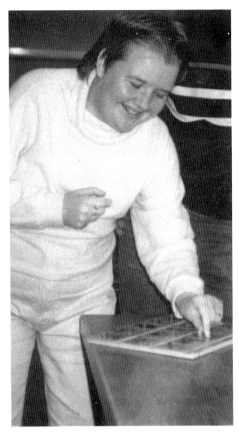

Fig. 5.2. Rett variant patient (S126) with partially preserved grasping ability. *(a)* Characteristic hand stereotypies. *(b)* Pincer grasping (after long latency of staring and hesitation).

Forme fruste RS may be considered in girls who show initially normal development followed by regression at age 1 to 3 years and in whom the developmental deviations are less prominent than in classical RS cases. Hand use may be partially preserved (Fig. 5.2). The classical RS hand stereotypies may be absent or atypical. The early skull (brain) growth deceleration may be so slight, and within the '–2SD range', as to be missed altogether. The summarized profile, course and pattern of RS abnormalities are usually less striking or complete, and yet, in retrospect at age 10 to 13 years, the diagnosis of RS seems indisputable. The deviations shown by forme fruste RS patients are more subtle both at initial presentation and later in childhood. During these early years, therefore, the majority of such patients are not suspected of having RS. Eventually, however, the convincing clusters of abnormalities and patterns of additional supporting RS manifestations develop.

The first recognized case of forme fruste RS was presented in 1985 at the Third

International Rett Syndrome Conference in Baltimore (Hagberg and Rasmussen 1986). The main details of that case are summarized here.

Case S48

This girl was born in 1968. She showed an uneventful pre-, peri- and neonatal history and completely normal development through her first 20 months of life. She then slowly lost acquired speech and developed several autistic traits. Her skull growth decelerated. There was mild dyspraxia. However, she did not completely stop using her hands, and the hand stereotypies characteristic of RS did not develop. Around age 4 years she slowly became more communicative again and also regained some of her previous fine motor skills and some speech. At age 17 years she showed most of the secondary abnormalities typical of adolescent girls with RS: acquired microcephaly, miniature abiotrophic feet, general growth retardation and scoliosis. She was moderately mentally retarded and could 'follow' a conversation, understanding simple instructions but showing severe difficulties performing tasks in spite of trying hard. Fine motor skills were impaired, but she could use her hands, even though a primitive pincer grasp prevailed. She had none of the characteristic RS hand stereotypies. However, she would pluck at her blouse in a stereotypic fashion, hands apart. She walked unsupported quite well but was unable to run, jump or stand on one leg. Neurological examination revealed dyspraxia and mild bilateral distal spasticity and peroneal muscle atrophy.

On follow-up at age 24 years she still showed fairly good gross motor performance and was even able to walk at a rather brisk pace. Sometimes, quite unexpectedly, she would speak single (even complicated) words. Hand dyspraxia was unchanged. She was highly insensitive to pain and would throw severe aggressive tantrums. Her scoliosis had not progressed, but she had developed a high kyphotic back profile.

Suzuki *et al.* (1986) confirmed the existence of incomplete forms of RS in two patients. One was a 7-year-old girl who lacked the characteristic hand stereotypies and could perform some purposeful hand movements, but who in other respects had the clinical developmental profile of RS. The other was a 19-year-old female who was able to run unsupported but who otherwise showed symptoms highly suggestive of RS.

In a questionnaire study to centres involved in RS research (Hagberg and Witt-Engerström 1986), about 20 cases of suspected forme fruste RS were reported.

Similar incomplete cases have recently been observed in Italy (Zappella 1992). In addition to a series of 102 classical RS patients evaluated over an eight-year period, Zappella, a child neuropsychiatrist with vast experience of RS behaviour patterns, has documented three atypical forme fruste patients with a remarkably well preserved ability to use grammatically correct phrase speech, but otherwise fulfilling most criteria for RS. One of these girls has a sister with classical RS.

From France, another atypical forme fruste patient with a phenotypically classical RS sister (early seizure onset variant) has been described (Journel *et al.* 1990). She was reported to have good understanding of many words. Both sisters and the mother in this family had a translocation of the X chromosome (Xp11.22).

The wide range of motor and other disabilities likely to exist in RS is amply demonstrated by recent results from twin studies. Kerr (1991, 1992), in Scotland, reported on a pair of monozygotic (MZ) twins identified in the course of the British Isles RS survey (cases BIS 197 and 198). The first-born (BIS 198) when examined at the age of 27 years was found to suffer from classical RS (stage IV). She was wheelchair dependent, with severe scoliosis and lower limb deformities. The second-born (BIS 197) seems, according to Kerr's description, to represent a forme fruste case. She was developmentally retarded and dyspraxic but with some preserved finger skills. She contributed to dressing herself and sang a few recognizable songs with word-like utterances.

In Yonago, Japan, in 1990 one of us (B.H.) had the opportunity to examine another MZ twin pair in the series (unpublished) of Takeshita and collaborators. The first twin (YM 7719) had fairly normal development until 18 months of age, but later lagged behind. At the age of 7¾ years this girl appeared to represent a case of 'simple' moderate mental retardation. Her gross and fine motor abilities were normal for her developmental level and she had none of the supporting symptoms and signs of RS. The second twin (KM 7718) had several RS characteristics and could best be described as a forme fruste variant. Development had appeared normal until about 12 months of age but then plateaued. Epilepsy appeared at age 1½ years. At 7¾ years she showed hand and gait dyspraxia and hand-clapping stereotypies of the RS type. There was a suspicion of mild lower limb spasticity, and communication was grossly deficient.

We have come across another variant of forme fruste in a 48-year-old woman (Case S116) with mild acquired dyspraxia plus other neurological signs. She had shown a sudden onset period of early regression and gradual development of acquired microcephaly. She is of particular interest because one of her sister's daughters has classical RS (Anvret et al. 1990). The case history is briefly summarized here.

Case S116
This woman was born in 1944. She had an uneventful early history. She learned to speak many single words, had good fine motor skills, crawled but could not walk unsupported at age 1 year. At that age she rapidly lost contact and communication ability, became shaky in the upright position and lost all finger skills. She became restless, agitated and severely mentally retarded. Some of her gross motor skills were later regained, but she never re-acquired fine motor skills and is still unable to eat with a spoon at the age of 48. She is now a small, severely mentally retarded woman with a peculiar behaviour pattern. She has cervical kyphosis, mild scoliosis and a small head. She communicates only through staring, as in classical cases of RS. Apart from severe hand dyspraxia, she also has gait dyspraxia with particular difficulties walking up and down stairs. There is no spasticity, dystonia or ataxia. She has well-controlled epilepsy (mixed type).

Preserved speech variant
One of the most characteristic features of classical RS is the loss of all acquired speech in the regression phase (stage II). However, some girls with RS who had acquired several words or even short phrases before regression at about age 2 years

will suddenly—and unexpectedly—utter one or more of these words quite distinctly several years later. The same words may be spoken again months or years later, usually in rather inappropriate situations, or they may never be heard again. This phenomenon has often been reported to occur in non-RS autism cases. The three forme fruste patients reported by Zappella (1992) and described above could also be considered to represent preserved speech variant cases.

Infantile seizure onset variant

The infantile seizure onset variant of RS—in which early onset seizures appear to 'blur' the characteristic onset symptomatology of RS—was first described by Hanefeld at the Second International Rett Syndrome Conference in Vienna, 1984 (Hanefeld 1985). He reported a girl with infantile spasms and hypsarrhythmia onset, who later developed classical RS (Hanefeld, personal communication). Early onset severe seizures (in one case reminiscent of infantile spasms) were also reported in two girls who later developed atypical variants of RS (Goutières and Aicardi 1986).

The Swedish RS series includes a girl (S70) who started having fits at 5½ months of age and went on to develop classical RS (with severe and, for a long time, therapy-resistant epilepsy) (Hagberg and Witt-Engerström 1987). In this case, reported below, there was familial epilepsy which appears to have set off the RS early, but blurred the phenotype during the first years of life. Three further cases with early seizure onset (one of whom had infantile spasms) were published by Maia *et al.* (1986). In the 1986 questionnaire study referred to above, we traced a dozen cases with the infantile seizure onset variant of RS (Hagberg and Witt-Engerström 1986). Since then several more cases have been diagnosed. In our own Swedish series from 1990 (Hagberg and Witt Engerström 1990*b*), seven out of 105 cases (6.7 per cent) had an onset with seizures at or under 6 months of age. In two of these seven cases, the characteristic RS presentation throughout stages I to III was definitely blurred by the epileptic disorder.

Case S70

This girl was born in 1984. She has a family history of seizures on the paternal side: several members have had cryptogenic epilepsy, febrile convulsions in infancy and childhood and other types of seizures. Her father, for instance, had a cryptogenic type of epilepsy throughout his childhood. A cousin, who is now quite healthy, had idiopathic infantile spasms with rapid treatment response.

The girl's own history was uneventful throughout pregnancy, delivery and the first five months of life. She then started having generalized fits (no infantile spasms, no EEG hypsarrhythmia) which, in conjunction with EEG abnormalities, were interpreted as postencephalitic, but which disappeared rapidly. Then, at age 8 months, she started having infantile spasms and was treated with ACTH. At that age she could no longer grasp objects and had lost her ability to sit up. There were then several months during which seizures of various types occurred and the EEG developed into continuous hypsarrhythmia. At age 2 years it was clear that she had significant head growth deceleration. RS-type hand-wringing had developed. Six months later she presented with fits of night laughter and breathing abnormalities of a panting type (without bloating). Her feet stopped growing and there were signs of autonomic dysfunction in the peripheral parts of her limbs. On follow-up at age 7 years 3 months she was severely motor disabled in a pattern characteristic of stage IV RS. There were severe breathing abnormalities with episodes of apnoea and Valsalva-type expiration. She also showed the type of bruxism which is typical of RS. There was complete apraxia and severe hypotonia with occasional dystonia. Kyphoscoliosis and subluxation of the left hip were also noted.

Case S75
This patient has been described in a previous publication (Gillberg 1989).

She was born in 1981. Caesarean section was performed because of signs of intrauterine asphyxia after 42 weeks gestation. The neonatal period was unremarkable. She was possibly a little late in all aspects of development, never very communicative, but acquired a few single words before age 15 months.

At 8 months she was noted to have a staring spell. This recurred at 16 months in combination with peripheral cyanosis and epileptogenic discharge on the EEG. This seizure, in retrospect, was the starting point for developmental regression and the appearance of severe autistic symptomatology. She was detached, destructive, showed stereotypic hand clapping and object flicking and would giggle (in the night as well as by day) for no obvious reason. At age 3 years she was diagnosed by one of us (C.G.) as having infantile autism and profound mental retardation. Only some years later was it apparent that she fitted the clinical picture of RS.

On follow-up at age 9 years she presented the classical picture of stage III RS. She had partial complex seizures at a rate of five to ten per day in spite of various antiepileptic medications. The EEG, which had previously shown a distinct sharp-wave focus in the posterior regions on the left side plus bilateral synchronous 3 to 4 Hz spike and wave activity in drowsiness, now showed a spike pattern centrotemporally in the right hemisphere. Single photon emission computerized tomography revealed considerable hypoperfusion in the left occipital parts of the right hemisphere and on the right side of the cerebellar hemisphere.

Our interpretation is that this girl, with otherwise classical RS, also contracted prenatally hypoxic–ischaemic brain damage on the right side. This might have blurred the clinical picture during the onset period and also complicated it through the stage II regression.

Also, among cases in the early seizure onset group, there have been interesting observations of marked phenotypic variation across twins in MZ pairs. In Belgium, Dr Erik Smeets showed one of us (B.H.) a 25-year-old woman (twin 1) with a history and features convincingly indicating a case of early stage IV RS. She had developed normally until 4 months of age, when infantile spasms and hypsarrhythmia occurred. She gradually developed RS, meeting most of the supportive criteria: irregular hyperventilation, screaming bursts, complete loss of fine motor functions, apraxia, ataxia, some dystonia and mild kyphoscoliosis. However, no skull growth deceleration had been documented. Twin 2 had the same early history with onset of infantile spasms at the age of 4 months. In addition, she had most of the RS-supporting symptomatology of her sister but in considerably milder degree. Her fine motor function in particular was far better than that of her co-twin, but she did not use her hands for practical purposes. Her stereotypies were mainly of the hand–tongue movement type and not of the classical RS pattern. Both twins are of small stature (145cm) and have bluish-red feet of normal size. Even if not meeting all RS criteria, the clinical picture is such that RS must be considered the most probable diagnosis, given that a lot of other possible diagnoses have been excluded over the years (Smeets, personal communication).

Congenital Rett syndrome
Congenital RS was first described by Rolando (1985). Her case 1, who at age 4 years showed all the clinical and EEG features of classical RS, was floppy and retarded from the very first months of life. Head control at 4 months was this girl's best gross motor skill. However, she apparently learned to reach for objects and to transfer them from one hand to the other. Her stage II regression period started at age 16 months when she became completely unresponsive with loss of all grasping skills.

It is now clear that, even though one of the diagnostic criteria for RS is 'apparently normal psychomotor development through the first six months', there are cases with otherwise classical RS symptoms but with mild, moderate or severe developmental deviations noted already in the first few months of life. Nomura had noted such mild developmental problems occurring from infancy in some RS girls as early as 1983 (Nomura *et al.* 1985). Al-Mateen *et al.* (1986) reported two girls with normal development to only age 4 months who then developed in a definitely abnormal fashion.

Goutières and Aicardi (1987) reported 14 patients with behavioural features suggestive of RS but failing to meet all the diagnostic criteria. In one of these girls (case 7) rapid deterioration might have occurred so early (at age 3 to 4 months) that previous development was rendered impossible to assess in retrospect. Another girl (case 8) in their series showed abnormally slow development from birth and deterioration during the period from 12 to 18 months, at which time epileptic fits occurred. Two of their other patients (cases 5 and 6) had abnormal development from birth, but later regression was questionable. Goutières and Aicardi concluded that these may be 'true' RS cases with an atypically early onset, or cases in which the period preceding the acquisition was not completely free of symptoms.

Recently, Lin *et al.* (1991) reported a girl (their case 6) with a similar clinical picture. She was retarded and hypotonic from birth. Her mother had observed reduced fetal movement during pregnancy. Infant development was slow. At age 12 months, generalized seizures appeared. She lost purposeful hand skills and her interest in the environment decreased. She then showed truncal ataxia, athetoid movements and decelerating skull growth. At age 4½ years acquired microcephaly was obvious.

Potential congenital RS cases were reported by Oguro *et al.* (1990) in their multi-institution survey of RS in Japan. Of 89 such patients identified, 54 were confirmed to have RS. In the other 35 cases the diagnosis remained questionable;

47

these patients had shown clinical signs of deterioration already in early infancy, had no characteristic RS stereotypies and were excluded from further evaluation because of an incomplete clinical picture.

We have come across similar borderline cases in our Swedish series, including the following girl, who was deviant already from birth but became more RS-like only as she approached school age.

Case S129
This girl is the third child of healthy parents who are first cousins. She was born after 38 weeks gestation. Delivery was uncomplicated and the birthweight and occipitofrontal circumference (OFC) were 3090g and 34cm respectively. She had feeding problems from the first day of life. She was floppy and appeared to be dull. At age 1 month she was constantly whining and screaming (including at night). At 2 months the parents still could not get gaze contact. At 6 months she was rather more hypotonic with considerable head lag. She showed no tendency to start grasping. At 10 months she had not progressed at all. However, after age 1 year she gradually began to be more alert and to develop with regard to motor skills. At 17 months she could roll over and sit unsupported. When seen by Dr Witt Engerström at age 23 months she was tentatively diagnosed as having an RS variant (congenital onset). She improved further and engaged in gaze and body contact. She was dyspraxic but was able to use a primitive opposed thumb–index finger grip. She babbled but ground her teeth. She had a stereotypic hand-clapping pattern. She had a marked dysequilibrium reaction and brisk lower limb tendon reflexes.

At age 6 years 3 months she appeared slightly malnourished and generally growth retarded with weight and height at the –2SD level. Her OFC was 49.5cm (and her skull growth curve showed a slight trend toward deceleration to –1SD). Her feet were disproportionately small. Severe constipation was a major problem. She showed stereotypic hand 'clapping' movements, usually with the hands not actually touching. There was clear fine and gross motor dyspraxia but no spasticity. She was unable to stand up and walk unsupported. Sleep was severely disturbed, with frequent awakenings and periods of night laughter. At age 7 years she is severely mentally retarded with many autistic traits. There is the type of intense staring gaze contact typical of RS. Extensive neurophysiological, neuro-imaging, cytogenetic and neurochemical investigations have yielded non-specific results.

This girl does not meet the main criteria for RS. Nevertheless, with increasing age her developmental profile and behavioural phenotype together provide support for the notion of a congenital onset RS variant.

Cases such as these demonstrate that the variation in RS phenotypes is probably considerably greater than originally anticipated. It is also clear that there is overlap between the various variants of RS, and that the borderlines between these are far from clear. For instance, our case S75 (see above), included in the section on 'infantile seizure onset RS', may not be widely discrepant from case 8 in the Goutières and Aicardi (1987) series, described in that paper as a possible example of 'congenital RS'.

Late childhood regression variants
Occasional cases of late childhood regression variants of RS have been reported in

which the clinical features through late infancy to early school age have clearly been those of 'simple' non-specific mental retardation with IQs in the low 50s to 40s. One of us (B.H.) coincidentally came across one such patient with an obvious RS phenotype at age 25 years, having previously examined her and excluded all classical RS criteria on several occasions between the ages of 3 years 8 months and 4 years 8 months. The medical and developmental history was confirmed by the mother—who was an astute observer—more than 20 years later. The main data from this case history are as follows.

Case S117

This woman was born in 1964 (after 37 weeks gestation) as the fourth child to healthy, unrelated parents. The pre- and perinatal histories were unrevealing. Already as a neonate she had a poor suck. She was floppy and developed a failure to thrive syndrome. Skull circumference data from early development are missing. She was late in communication and did not babble like other infants in late infancy. She sat (but could not sit up) at age 8 months and walked unsupported at age 13 months. She eventually learned to run. She developed a pincer grasp and was able to eat with a spoon early on. She learned some single words from age 2 to 3 years but still had no phrase-speech by age 4 years 8 months. At that time she nevertheless had good contact with her parents, played with her doll (giving it food to eat with a spoon) and could ride on a tricycle. She was diagnosed as having moderate mental retardation without any signs of ataxia, spasticity or dyskinesia.

From age 7 years she gradually lost acquired speech and fine motor skills. She deteriorated in general behaviour and overall performance.

When seen at age 25 years she was small (152cm) with a proportionately small head (52cm) and kyphoscoliosis. Her abdomen was distended and she had a bloating habit. She showed stereotypic general motor activity, walking around in circles on the floor, hands clasped together. At rest, she continuously performed Rett-like plucking and scratching movements with the right hand on the back of the left, the hands being held more loosely together. She had marked dyspraxia but would suddenly grab things unexpectedly. She had lower motor neuron impairment with distal limb atrophy and pes cavus, also decreased awareness of pain and sudden bouts of unprovoked screaming and laughter. In addition, staff at the hostel where she was staying provided convincing details about this woman's power of observation and her ability to absorb information and to communicate her needs by intense gazing and 'eye pointing'.

We have also come across another case possibly representing a late childhood regression RS variant.

Case S120

This case has been described in more detail in a previous publication (Gillberg 1989).

This woman was born in 1962. She was the second girl born to healthy and unrelated parents. Pregnancy, delivery and the neonatal period were uneventful. During the first 10 months of life there was nothing noticeably wrong about her development, but it then became apparent that she was a little slow in gross motor development. She had a well-developed pincer grip at age 14 months and walked unsupported at 18 months. At 19 months she had a high temperature and a sore throat and thereafter became hyperactive, restless and irritable, with screaming and autistic traits. A year later she was diagnosed as having

49

infantile autism and moderate mental retardation. In retrospect it is obvious that the clinical picture, except for the time of onset, was very much that of disintegrative psychosis (Evans-Jones and Rosenbloom 1978).

At age 8 years she rather quickly developed severe scoliosis which was operated on when she was 12 years old. She remained autistic throughout childhood but became less hyperactive with time.

Symptoms compatible with a diagnosis of RS gradually developed from middle to late childhood. When seen at age 22 years she was still severely autistic, but otherwise fitted the clinical picture of RS in many ways. She showed intense hand-washing stereotypies in the midline which developed after a gradual deterioration of fine motor skills throughout school age. She would not use her hands for anything except stereotypies unless forced to, and then grabbing only very clumsily. Her hands and feet were small and cold. She had passed puberty. On the Vineland Social Maturity Scale (Doll 1965) she functioned in the lowest range of the severe mental retardation spectrum. She had staring spells, and her EEG pattern was highly suggestive of RS.

At follow-up at age 30 she is a small (150cm), intensely staring, immature woman with girl-like features, still mobile (stage III) but with gait dyspraxia. The neurological abnormalities consist of combined dyspraxia, ataxia and mild lower limb spasticity. In addition she has obvious lower motor neuron impairment, pes cavus and trophic changes. Interestingly, she is now communicating surprisingly well with her parents, and they confirm a slowly improving level of contact and communication. Moreover, she has learned to eat with a spoon and to drink from a glass. This woman has never had any epileptic manifestations.

What makes this case deviate from the picture of classical RS are the onset and course of the disorder, the relatively normal head circumference (OFC 52cm) and the lack of information on decelerating skull growth. She also has only some of the supporting RS manifestations. Nevertheless, the clinical profile and the cluster of symptoms and signs convincingly indicate a variant of RS.

Clusters of familial atypical variants

There have been about a dozen familial cases of RS in the literature, not counting the seven pairs of MZ concordant twins which have been reported to date (Ellison *et al.* 1992).

No doubt there are families with more than two potential RS candidates and with marked differences in patterns of developmental deviation across family members. Gillberg *et al.* (1990) described a family in which three female maternal cousins presented with severe developmental/neuropsychiatric disorder. Case C in that study had classical RS (case S36 in the comprehensive Swedish series). Case B had infantile autism, mild mental retardation and (truncal and gait) ataxia, which improved with age. Case A was diagnosed as having infantile autism and profound mental retardation. Interestingly, at adolescence this girl started 'washing' her hands in the midline in an RS-like fashion, and long before that she had shown midline hand-clapping. She was also extremely obese and showed the type of abnormal eating behaviour typical of Prader–Willi syndrome. This may be particularly relevant given the recent description of RS-like symptoms in some female patients with Angelman syndrome (which like Prader–Willi syndrome maps to the q11–13 portion of chromosome 15) and in some males with a 15q11–13 marker chromosome syndrome (see below).

Monozygotic twin variability

The remarkable phenotypical variability of some MZ twins was described in the sections on forme fruste and early seizure onset RS variants. In fact, when surveying the published reports on MZ twins, phenotypical concordance seems to be the exception rather than the rule.

To give an example of this, the set of MZ twins described by Coleman *et al.* (1987) developed RS at a slightly different rate with clinical dissimilarities. For instance, one was a typical looking, thin RS child who showed hand wringing in the midline, while the other was slightly plump and showed no typical RS stereotypies. This latter twin showed signs of spasticity such as bilateral fisting and crossed ankles whereas the former had neither. The paternal family history included a mentally retarded great-grandmother, two of whose daughters had progressive retardation and died before age 25 years.

General comments on the phenotypical variability in Rett syndrome girls

Over the past few years it has become clear that the RS phenotype is much more variable than originally believed. Some case reports suggest, albeit indirectly, that there may even be females with unexplained 'simple' or 'uncomplicated' mental retardation who, in the end, will turn out to have the same biological abnormality that underlies classical RS. This makes the need to find a diagnostic marker mandatory. In the search for such a marker we need to concentrate on the narrowly defined nucleus group with classical RS. This does not mean that we should ignore all the possible variants, which in themselves could contribute to finding the marker. However, we need to define *exactly* which groups are being studied, or we may end up on the wrong biological road.

Rettoid males

Only a handful of syndromes in medicine have been described which occur exclusively (or almost exclusively) in females.

There are, of course, the syndromes attributable to sex chromosome aneuploidies, such as Turner syndrome (XO) and triple X syndrome (XXX), which, for obvious reasons, can only occur in females. However, no consistent chromosomal aberration, structural or numerical, has been documented in Rett syndrome.

A few other rare syndromes, such as orofaciodigital syndrome, Goltz syndrome (focal dermal hypoplasia) and incontinentia pigmenti have been convincingly documented in females only. However, all these syndromes are believed to be inherited in a dominant fashion and are possibly lethal in the male.

Such a mode of inheritance does not appear to be operating in RS (see Chapter 10).

Some clearly X-linked disorders, such as haemophilia A, produce severe symptoms in males only. Otherwise, in the male, there are no obvious counterparts to the apparent sex exclusiveness seen in RS.

In the early 1980s, an hypothesis linking RS with a two-step mutation on the X chromosomes was proposed. According to this hypothesis, a heritable mutation on one of the X chromosomes would be required together with an added non-heritable mutation on the other X chromosome. No firm evidence in support of this hypothesis has been gained so far (Anvret and Wahlström 1992). If this were indeed the aetiology of RS, one would not expect to find males with a normal karyotype and RS (who, if they had the heritable X chromosome mutation, might be expected not to survive *in utero*). However, RS could occur in a male with the Klinefelter syndrome (XXY). So far, no case report linking RS with the XXY abnormality has been published.

No indisputable cases of RS in the male have appeared in the literature to date, even though a number of authors have described Rettoid males (Gillberg 1989, Coleman 1990, Eeg-Olofsson *et al.* 1990, Philippart 1990, Topçu *et al.* 1991). These Rettoid males meet some but not all of the necessary criteria for Rett syndrome. (The patient reported by Eeg-Olofsson *et al.* was said to meet all the diagnostic criteria, but the clinical description in the published paper is not sufficiently detailed to allow definite conclusions in this respect.) Could it be that the RS phenotype is different (slightly or considerably) in males than in females? Theoretically this would not seem unreasonable, even though it does seem *unlikely* given the lack of counterparts to such a sex-linked skewing of symptomatology in the rest of developmental medicine or neuropsychiatry. In the fragile X syndrome, there appear to be clear differences between males and females (Hagerman 1989). However, some differences would be expected given the sex-linked genetic aberration demonstrated in this syndrome (Gillberg and Coleman 1992). Nevertheless, it is slightly puzzling that exactly the same type of severe symptomatology (autism, hyperactivity and severe mental retardation) occurs in fragile X positive females as in fragile X positive males, even though the proportion with severe symptoms is much smaller in females. Also, there appear to be some *developmental differences* between the sexes in the fragile X syndrome even when the target symptoms in a cross-sectional study are the same (Gillberg and Coleman 1992). There are a number of other developmental/neuropsychiatric syndromes that are considerably more common in males than in females (*e.g.* autism, Tourette syndrome and dyslexia). However, the evidence so far is that the male and female phenotypes in these disorders do not show any clear differences.

In summary, on the basis of the published evidence RS appears to be unique in that it occurs in classical form in females only.

In the following, we describe two males with Rettoid symptomatology seen by ourselves. These two cases, together with the other four cases in the literature, are summarized in Table 5.2.

Case M1

This boy was born in 1980, the first-born child of unrelated parents. Delivery was by caesarean section in the 38th week of gestation following moderate toxaemia during the previous month of pregnancy. The mother was treated with terbutaline throughout pregnancy because of asthma. Toward the end of pregnancy she was also given hydralazine and metoprolol for high blood pressure. Birthweight and length were 3150g and 49cm respectively. He had moderate asphyxia (Apgar scores 4 and 5 at 1 and 5 minutes), neonatal breathing difficulties and slight hyperbilirubinaemia (max. 270mmol/L), and he received oxygen treatment (at 45 per cent) and light therapy.

He was probably never normal and showed some minor physical anomalies (bilateral epicanthal folds, slight hypertelorism and low-set ears). His growth was normal (50th centile for OFC, 10th centile for height and weight) until about the age of 6 months. From then there was OFC deceleration down to the 3rd centile at age 2 years. General growth stunting also occurred and he was at or below the 1st centile already by age 1 year. From around age 6 to 8 months the parents noted severe autistic withdrawal and lack of communication. It is unclear whether some of these symptoms (or antecedents) were present before that date. Clinical work-up revealed a cytomegalovirus (CMV) infection, but it was not possible to establish whether this was congenital or had been acquired after birth. From around age 3 years he developed staring spells and epilepsy was diagnosed. His EEG was grossly abnormal (see below). His hands and feet were noted to be very cold. Severe feeding difficulties were observed already at this age.

When seen for neuropsychiatric evaluation at ages 9, 10 and 11 years he showed the following features: general growth retardation (height at age 10.3 years, 115cm; weight, 18kg; OFC, 51cm), minor physical facial anomalies as above, marked but short-curved thoracic scoliosis, cold feet and hands, little hand-use and reluctance to use hands for purposeful activities, hand stereotypies of various kinds, often in the midline and often of the wringing 'Rettoid' type. His neuroimpairments were: ataxic gait and mild truncal ataxia, staring (epileptic) spells, autistic behaviour (scoring 90 on the Autism Behavior Checklist (ABC) at age 10), abnormal non-verbal communication but periods of intense gaze contact, no speech and profound mental retardation. He also had enlarged external genitalia with hyperpigmentation of the genital region.

The EEG had shown slowing of the background rhythm in the lateral frontal regions on the left side and diffuse occurrence of episodic spikes and waves during sleep when the patient was 4 years of age, but was later normal on several occasions (during antiepileptic treatment). It did not conform with the characteristic RS pattern and development. Chromosomal culture (including in a folic acid depleted medium) at age 11 years was normal. Extensive laboratory examinations were unrevealing. Mucopolysaccharidosis and oligosaccharidosis were convincingly excluded.

In summary, this boy showed several of the symptoms of RS including OFC deceleration, growth stunting, loss of some hand skills, typical hand stereotypies, peripheral vasomotor disturbance, constipation and scoliosis. He met six of the nine necessary criteria and six of the eight supportive criteria for RS as defined by the Rett Syndrome Diagnostic Criteria Work Group (Trevathan *et al.* 1988). He also met criteria for autistic disorder (see Table 5.2). Nevertheless, the overall clinical impression was not that of RS. No clear aetiology could be established, but he did have a CMV infection before 6 months of age.

Case M2

This boy has been described in two previous publications (Gillberg and Winnergård 1984, Gillberg 1989).

TABLE 5.2

Diagnostic criteria for Rett syndrome and autistic disorder met by males in case reports in the literature

Criterion	Cases meeting criterion†
Necessary criteria for Rett syndrome[1]	
(1) Apparently normal pre- and perinatal period	4,5,6
(2) Apparently normal psychomotor development through first 6 months	3,4,5,7
(3) Normal head circumference at birth	1,2
(4) Deceleration of head growth between ages 6 months and 4 years	1,2,5
(5) Loss of purposeful hand use between ages 6 and 30 months, temporally associated with communication dysfunction and social withdrawal	1*,2*,3,4,5,6**,7**
(6) Development of severely impaired expressive and receptive language, and presence of apparent severe psychomotor retardation	1,2,3,4,5,6,7?
(7) Stereotypic hand movements (of Rettoid type)	1,2,3,4,5,6,7
(8) Appearance of gait apraxia and/or truncal ataxia between ages 1 and 4 years	1,2,3,4,5,6,7
(9) Diagnosis tentative until 2–5 years of age	1,2,3,7
Supportive criteria for Rett syndrome	
(1) Breathing dysfunction	2,4,5
(2) EEG abnormalities	1,5,6**
(3) Seizures	1,2,4,5,6
(4) Spasticity, muscle wasting, dystonia	4,5,6,7
(5) Peripheral vasomotor disturbance	1,2,3,4
(6) Scoliosis	1,2,4,5,6
(7) Growth retardation	1,2,3,4,5,6
(8) Hypotrophic small feet	1,2,4,5

Exclusion criteria for Rett syndrome
Not clearly met, although case 1 had CMV infection identified before 6 months of age and case 2 had Moebius syndrome diagnosed early in life. There was extrauterine asphyxia in cases 1, 2 and 3 at birth, but there was no clear evidence that this led to brain damage. There was evidence of intrauterine growth retardation in case 4. There were insufficient data in cases 6 and 7 to judge whether exclusion criteria applied or not →

He was born in 1979 and is the only child of unrelated healthy parents. He was born after 42 weeks gestation and had severe but brief extrauterine asphyxia. He was suspected of having Moebius syndrome at a few months of age because of sucking difficulties and poor mimicry. However, this diagnosis was not made with confidence until he was 25 months old. Developmental delay and deviance were not clearly suspected before 30 months of age. His head circumference decelerated from the 60th centile at 22 months (49.5cm) to the 10th centile at 13 years (50.5cm).

He started walking unsupported at 2 years and developed favourably with regard to gross motor skills for the next three years. Truncal ataxia and a broad-based gait have since become more and more obvious. At 2½ to 3 years autistic symptoms appeared. He became withdrawn, using the phrase-speech he had acquired only in a parrot-like echoing fashion. From around age 3 to 3½ years there was an apparent set-back during which he lost some of his communication skills and seemed puzzled and lacking in initiative. At 5 years he was referred for symptoms of autism to an autism treatment centre, where he has been followed by one of us for many years. From around age 2½ years he has hyperventilated and intermittently held his breath.

Criteria for autistic disorder (DSM-III-R)[2]	Case M1	Case M2
Qualitative impairment in reciprocal social interaction:		
(1) lack of awareness of others	√	√
(2) no seeking of comfort	√	√
(3) no or impaired imitation	√	√
(4) no or abnormal social play	√	√
(5) gross impairment in ability to make peer friendships	√	√
Qualitative impairment in communication and imaginative activity:		
(6) no mode of communication	√	√
(7) abnormal non-verbal communication	√	√
(8) absence of imaginative activity	√	√
(9) marked abnormalities in production of speech		√
(10) marked abnormalities in form or content of speech		
(11) marked impairment in ability to converse despite adequate speech		
Markedly restricted repertoire of activities and interests		
(12) stereotypies	√	√
(13) persistent preoccupation with parts of objects	√	√
(14) marked distress over trivial changes in environment		√
(15) insistence on routines	√	√
(16) markedly restricted range of interests		
Onset during infancy or childhood		√
Number of criteria for autistic disorder met (excluding onset criterion)	10	13

*There does not appear to have been complete loss of purposeful hand movements in either of these boys, but both showed a gradual decrease in hand use for a long period some time during the first 7 years of life.

**Insufficient data to judge to what extent this symptom applied.

†Cases 1,2—this Chapter; 3—Coleman (1990); 4,5—Philippart (1990); 6—Eeg-Olofsson *et al.* (1990); 7—Topçu *et al.* (1991).

[1]See Table 2.1 (p. 8).

[2]American Psychiatric Association (1987).

At age 13 years he shows extreme bloating with severe distension of the abdomen. It is difficult to get him to eat and he is constantly constipated. His hands and feet are small and cold. He is generally extremely small, the size of a 5-year old. His Griffiths developmental quotient, 69 at age 4.8 years, was only 49 at age 9.6 years despite intensive behavioural treatment, social training and special education. From around age 6 years he has shown staring spells, although at that age his EEG was normal. He has midline hand stereotypies of the RS type, but also has other types of hand stereotypy (waving, finger flicking, etc.). When young he had excellent fine motor skills, and at 5 years he could manipulate small objects with considerable precision. Over the last eight years he has shown a gradual decrease in hand use such that he can no longer eat with a spoon and can only just drink out of a mug if given much physical support. However, as late as at age 11 years he could still perform well with his hands for very brief periods (of 10 to 15 seconds) if highly motivated, 'excited' or prompted. Gradually he has become more dyspraxic. He often stands 'frozen' in the middle of a room as though he does not know how to get out of there. If pushed slightly he starts walking but then becomes 'frozen' again.

He has developed a slowly progressive thoracic scoliosis.

In summary, this boy would have been considered for a diagnosis of RS had he not been diagnosed as having Moebius syndrome and had he not been male. He showed OFC deceleration, growth stunting, loss of some hand skills, typical hand stereotypies, truncal and gait ataxia, general apraxia, hyperventilation, breath-holding spells, peripheral vasomotor disturbance, constipation and scoliosis. He met six of the nine necessary and six of the eight supportive criteria for RS.

For both of these boys a case could be made for diagnosing both autism and RS. Neither meet all the classical criteria for RS, but both correspond to the description of autistic disorder in the DSM-III-R (American Psychiatric Association 1987). Autism, in recent years, has been shown to be a behavioural disorder with a multitude of different aetiologies (Gillberg and Coleman 1992). In the end, RS could also turn out to be a syndrome of multiple aetiologies.

The two male cases described above, together with the four others reported in the literature, illustrate that there are males who have many features suggestive of RS. We submit that these may be 'Rettoid' cases rather than examples of true RS. As far as we are aware, no male patient meeting all the criteria for RS has yet been described. Nevertheless, these cases are sufficiently similar to some of the forme fruste and Rett variant cases encountered in females to warrant a cautious attitude when dismissing the notion of RS in males. No clear aetiology has been established for any of the male cases, and eventually some of them may be shown to have the same diagnostic marker which may be demonstrated for RS in females. Equally possible, however, is the association of male Rettoid cases with other and variable aetiologies. There is clearly Rettoid symptomatology in a number of other developmental/neuropsychiatric conditions (see below).

Several traits (RS-type stereotypies, ataxia, little hand use after a period of regression, epilepsy, breathing dysfunction, small hands and feet and unprovoked laughter) reminiscent both of RS and Angelman syndrome have been documented in a number of boys with a marker chromosome abnormality involving the q11–13 segment of chromosome 15 (Gillberg *et al.* 1991). In all such cases examined by us, this defect has been inherited from the (healthy) mother. RS-type hand-washing/hand-wringing has also been observed in males with autism associated with Moebius syndrome and even in some with tuberous sclerosis (Gillberg 1992). This symptomatic overlap could indicate genetic overlap, but might equally demonstrate that 'pathognomonic' RS symptoms may be highly non-specific.

Summing up, we have not been able to find unequivocal evidence that RS in males exists. However, this should not detract from the possibility that RS may ultimately be shown to be a condition without the exclusive association with the female sex supposed/suggested today.

Rett-like symptoms in other known syndromes
During the past few years it has become obvious that many of the symptoms encountered in RS are sometimes seen in other syndromes as well. For instance, the hand-washing stereotypies once believed to be specific to RS are seen in several

widely discrepant conditions (Gillberg 1992). Only the remarkable and substantial loss of acquired purposeful hand skills appears to differentiate RS, but incomplete loss of such skills is probably also present in a number of other severe developmental/neuropsychiatric conditions.

In clinical practice, the syndromes most often causing diagnostic confusion are (1) non-RS idiopathic autism, (2) infantile neuronal ceroid lipofuscinosis, and (3) Angelman syndrome. Several Rett-like symptoms are also frequently encountered in the 15q11–13 marker chromosome syndrome described by Gillberg *et al.* (1991), occasionally in Moebius syndrome and rarely in fragile X positive girls.

Non-RS idiopathic variants of autism can often not be clearly distinguished from RS in the very early stages of the disorder, even though claims for distinguishing features in infancy have been made (Olsson and Rett 1985, Gillberg 1987). The course of the disorder will eventually turn out to be different, though, and a distinction should be possible around age 2 to 3 years in most cases. However, it is appropriate to point out that a diagnosis of RS does not exclude a diagnosis of autism and vice versa. Autism, like epilepsy, is only a descriptive term for a set of symptoms and not an aetiological diagnostic label.

Infantile neuronal ceroid lipofuscinosis (INCL), which is considerably less common than RS, in its early stages can be virtually indistinguishable from stage II RS. Clinically, the differential diagnosis is extremely problematic in the age period from 15 to 30 months. After age 3 years the two conditions diverge considerably (Hagberg and Witt-Engerström 1990*a*). Early findings of cortical atrophy on CT scan and a suppressed flattened EEG should give suspicion. INCL can be differentiated by ultramicroscopy at skin biopsy and through DNA gene technology. INCL maps to the short arm of chromosome 1 (Järvelä *et al.* 1991).

We have seen the *Angelman syndrome* in two girls for whom the referral diagnosis was 'RS?'. In both cases there was severe mental retardation, ataxia, complete muteness, some hand dyspraxia and midline hand stereotypies and epilepsy. Night and daytime bursts of unprovoked laughter also occurred. We have demonstrated the 15q11–13 Angleman chromosomal defect in one of these cases (personal data, unpublished). In contrast to RS girls, those with Angelman syndrome have global developmental delay from early infancy and there is no clear loss of acquired skills nor deceleration of skull growth, but usually early onset epilepsy with characteristic EEG changes (Robb *et al.* 1989).

In some girls with the *fragile X syndrome*, differential diagnostic problems may arise in relation to RS. Such problems would seem to be relevant only in the very young age group. Autistic-like features, night laughter and bruxism in combination with motor and mental retardation in the 1- to 2-year-old age range can lead to the suspicion of an atypical variant of RS. However, after age 2 years, diagnosis is usually not difficult. Again, one important differentiating feature is the remarkable loss of acquired fine motor skills in RS which is not present in the fragile X syndrome.

Final remarks

It is evident that RS is a considerably broader and more complex concept than was supposed from the original reports (Rett 1966, Hagberg *et al.* 1983). Nevertheless, given the present clinical boundaries it continues to appear likely that it affects exclusively females. A boy with an RS-like phenotype should never be considered for a diagnosis of RS unless an extensive neuroimaging, biochemical and cytogenetic work-up has been performed. For a preschool girl with a classic set of necessary and supporting criteria, the diagnostic work-up may be less extensive: a cytogenetic mapping including examination for fragile X, an EEG as a starting point for later follow-up, a CT of the brain, and standard urinary screening examinations for patterns of amino acids, organic acids, mucopolysaccharides and oligosaccharides. To trace girls likely to have RS but presenting with phenotypes outside the classical RS nucleus group is difficult. Clinical experience, a high degree of 'sensitivity' to developmental history, and systematic follow-up, sometimes for years, will provide the best hints. If the concept of RS as a whole syndrome of several clinical variants is correct, then RS may turn out to be the second most important single disease entity (next to Down syndrome) underlying severe mental retardation in the female sex.

ACKNOWLEDGEMENTS

The studies were supported by grants from the following foundations: Vera and Hans Albrechtson, Gunnar and Märtha Bergendahl, Frimurare-Barnhusdirektionen, Sunnerdahl and W:6 Rett Research.

REFERENCES

Al-Mateen, M., Philippart, M., Shields, W.D. (1986) 'Rett syndrome: a commonly overlooked progressive encephalopathy in girls.' *American Journal of Disabled Children*, **140**, 761–765.

American Psychiatric Association (1987) *Diagnostic and Statistical Manual of Mental Disorders. 3rd Edn—Revised.* Washington, DC: APA.

Anvret, M., Wahlström, J. (1992) 'Genetics of the Rett syndrome.' *Brain and Development*, **14** (Suppl.), S101–S103.

—— —— Skogsberg, P., Hagberg, B. (1990) 'Segregation analysis of the X-chromosome in a family with Rett syndrome in two generations.' *American Journal of Medical Genetics*, **37**, 31–35.

Coleman, M. (1990) 'Is classical Rett syndrome ever present in males?' *Brain and Development*, **12**, 31–32.

—— Naidu, S., Murphy, M., Pines, M., Bias, W. (1987) 'A set of monozygotic twins with Rett syndrome.' *Brain and Development*, **9**, 475–478.

Doll, E. (1965) *Vineland Social Maturity Scale. Revised Edition.* Circle Pines, MN: American Guidance Service.

Eeg-Olofsson, O., Al-Zuhair, A.G.H., Teebi, A.S., Zaki, M., Daoud, A.S. (1990) 'A boy with the Rett syndrome?' *Brain and Development*, **12**, 529–532.

Ellison, K.A., Fill, C.P., Terwilliger, J., DeGennaro, L.J., Martin-Gallardo, A., Anvret, M., Percy, A.K., Ott, J., Zoghbi, H. (1992) 'Examination of X chromosome markers in Rett syndrome: Exclusion mapping with a novel variation on multilocus linkage analysis.' *American Journal of Medical Genetics*, **50**, 278–287.

Evans-Jones, L.G., Rosenbloom, L. (1978) 'Disintegrative psychoses in childhood.' *Developmental Medicine and Child Neurology*, **20**, 462–470.

Gillberg, C. (1987) 'Autistic symptoms in Rett syndrome: the first two years according to mother reports.' *Brain and Development*, **9**, 499–501.

—— (1989) 'The borderland of autism and Rett syndrome: five case histories to highlight diagnostic difficulties.' *Journal of Autism and Developmental Disorders*, **19**, 545–559.

—— (1992) 'The Emanuel Miller Lecture 1991: Autism and autistic-like conditions. Subgroups of disorders of empathy.' *Journal of Child Psychology and Psychiatry*, **33**, 813–842.

—— Coleman, M. (1992) *The Biology of the Autistic Syndromes. 2nd Edn. Clinics in Developmental Medicine No. 126.* London: Mac Keith Press with Cambridge University Press.

—— Winnergård, I. (1984) 'Childhood psychosis in a case of Moebius syndrome.' *Neuropediatrics*, **15**, 147–149.

—— Ehlers, S., Wahlström, J. (1990) 'The syndromes described by Kanner and Rett–Hagberg: overlap in an extended family.' *Developmental Medicine and Child Neurology*, **32**, 258–261.

—— Steffenburg, S., Wahlström, J., Gillberg, I.C., Sjöstedt, A., Martinsson, T., Liedgren, S., Eeg-Olofsson, O. (1991) 'Case study: Autism associated with marker chromosome.' *Journal of the American Academy of Child and Adolescent Psychiatry*, **30**, 489–494.

Goutières, F., Aicardi, J. (1986) 'Atypical forms of Rett syndrome.' *American Journal of Medical Genetics*, **24** (Suppl. 1), 183–194.

—— —— (1987) 'New experience with Rett syndrome in France: The problem of atypical cases.' *Brain and Development*, **9**, 502–505.

Hagberg, B., Rasmussen, P. (1986) '"Forme fruste" of Rett syndrome—a case report.' *American Journal of Medical Genetics*, **24** (Suppl. 1), 175–181.

—— Witt-Engerström, I. (1986) 'Rett syndrome: A suggested staging system for describing impairment profile with increasing age towards adolescence.' *American Journal of Medical Genetics*, **24** (Suppl. 1), 47–59.

—— —— (1987) 'Rett syndrome: epidemiology and nosology—progress in knowledge 1986.' *Brain and Development*, **9**, 451–457.

—— —— (1990*a*) 'Early stages of the Rett syndrome and infantile neuronal ceroid lipofuscinosis—a difficult differential diagnosis.' *Brain and Development*, **12**, 20–22.

—— —— (1990*b*) 'Swedish Rett syndrome basic data register 1960–90.' *Acta Paediatrica Scandinavica*, Suppl. 369, 43–54. *(Appendix.)*

—— Goutières, F., Hanefeld, F., Rett, A., Wilson, J. (1985) 'Rett syndrome: criteria for inclusion and exclusion.' *Brain and Development*, **7**, 372–373.

—— Aicardi, J., Dias, K., Ramos, O. (1983) 'A progressive syndrome of autism, dementia, ataxia, and loss of purposeful hand use in girls: Rett's syndrome: Report of 35 cases.' *Annals of Neurology*, **14**, 471–479.

Hagerman, R.J. (1989) 'Chromosomes, genes and autism.' *In:* Gillberg, C. (Ed.) *Diagnosis and Treatment of Autism.* New York: Plenum.

Hanefeld, F. (1985) 'The clinical pattern of the Rett syndrome.' *Brain and Development*, **7**, 320–325.

Journel, H., Melki, J., Turleau, C., Munnich, A., de Grouchy, J. (1990) 'Rett phenotype with X/autosome translocation: Possible mapping to the short arm of chromosome X.' *American Journal of Medical Genetics*, **35**, 142–147.

Järvelä, I., Schleutker, J., Haataja, L., Santavuori, P., Puhakka, L., Manninen, T., Palotie, A., Sandkuijl, L.A., Renlund, M., White, R., et al. (1991) 'Infantile form of neuronal ceroid lipofuscinosis (CLNI) maps to the short arm of chromosome 1.' *Genomics*, **9**, 170–173.

Kerr, A. (1991) 'Twins with Rett syndrome.' *Paper presented at the 2nd World Congress on Psychiatric Genetics, Glasgow.*

—— (1992) 'British longitudinal study (1982–1991) and 1990 survey.' *Paper presented at the 1st European Congress on Mental Retardation and Medical Care, April 1991, Noordwijkerhout, The Netherlands.*

Lin, M-Y., Wang, P-J., Lin, L-H., Shen, Y Z. (1991) 'The Rett and Rett-like syndromes: A broad concept.' *Brain and Development*, **13**, 228–231.

Maia, M., Barbot, C., Barbosa, C., Alves, D., Bothelo, B. (1986) 'Syndrome de Rett et ses limites: à propos de 15 cas.' *Report to the French sector meeting of the European Federation of Child Neurology Societies, Paris.*

Nomura, Y., Segawa, M., Hasegawa, M. (1985) 'Rett syndrome—an early catecholamine and indolamine deficient disorder?' *Brain and Development*, **7**, 334–341.

Oguro, N., Momoi, M., Nakamigawa, T., Miyamoto, S., Kobayashi, S., Miyao, M., Kamoshita, S. (1990) 'Multi-institutional survey of the Rett syndrome in Japan.' *Brain and Development*, **12**, 753–759.

Olsson, B., Rett, A. (1985) 'Behavioural observations concerning differential diagnosis between Rett syndrome and autism.' *Brain and Development*, 7, 281–289.

Philippart, M. (1990) 'The Rett syndrome in males.' *Brain and Development*, 12, 33–36.

Rett, A. (1966) *Über ein cerebral-atrophisches Syndrom bei Hyperammonämie*. Vienna: Brüder Hollinek.

Robb, S.A., Pohl, K.R.E., Baraitser, M., Wilson, J., Brett, E.M. (1989) 'The 'happy puppet' syndrome of Angelman. Review of the clinical features.' *Archives of Disease in Childhood*, 64, 83–86.

Rolando, S. (1985) 'Rett syndrome: Report of eight cases.' *Brain and Development*, 7, 290–296.

Rossiter, E.J.R., Callaghan, C. (1987) 'Rett's syndrome in an Australian girl.' *Australia and New Zealand Journal of Developmental Disabilities*, 13, 201–209.

Suzuki, H., Matsouka, T., Hiriyama, Y., Sakuragawa, N., Arima, M., Tateno, A., Tojo, M., Suzuki, V. (1986) 'Rett syndrome: Progression of symptoms from infancy to childhood.' *Journal of Child Neurology*, 1, 137–141.

Topçu, M., Topaloğlu, H., Renda, Y., Berker, M., Turanli, G. (1991) 'The Rett syndrome in males.' *Brain and Development*, 13, 62. *(Letter.)*

Trevathan, E., Moser, H.W., Opitz, J.M., Percy, A.K., Naidu, S., Holm, V.A., Boring, C.C., Janssen, R.S., Yeargin-Allsopp, M., Adams, M.J., *et al.* (1988) 'Diagnostic criteria for Rett syndrome. The Rett Syndrome Diagnostic Criteria Work Group.' *Annals of Neurology*, 23, 425–428.

Zappella, M. (1992) 'The Rett girls with preserved speech.' *Brain and Development*, 14, 98–101.

6
SCOLIOSIS IN RETT SYNDROME

Eira Stokland, Jan Lidström and Bengt Hagberg

Progressive scoliosis is an important problem for the majority of RS females (Hagberg *et al.* 1983, Naidu *et al.* 1986). In a recent extensive questionnaire study, Bassett and Tolo (1990) showed that two thirds of 11- to 15-year old RS girls (mean 12¼ years) had developed a spinal deformity. Naidu *et al.* (1986) observed more rapid progression of scoliosis in non-ambulatory RS patients. Swedish data from 30 adult RS women aged 22 to 44 years (median 27 years) (Witt-Engerström and Hagberg 1990) revealed that no less than 22 had a significant curvature, all but two of whom were in the non-ambulant stage IV of RS in the clinical classification introduced by Hagberg and Witt-Engerström (1986). Moreover, those who had never been able to walk (Stage IV-B) had in all cases developed their scoliosis in early school age (Witt Engerström 1990), and in most it was severely disabling, preventing normal sitting.

In this chapter we report a survey, based on the Swedish clinical RS series (see Chapter 3), of spinal deformities and their relation to clinical stage, severity of disease and age. In addition we discuss predisposing types of neuroimpairment, pathophysiology and guidelines for clinical management.

Materials and methods
I. General neuropaediatric study
From the Swedish RS series of 106 patients with classical and forme fruste RS, data from 76, with satisfactory clinical examination protocols, were used: 29 with retrospective data from the age period 11 to 15 years (Group A) and 47 with evaluations at age 18 years or later (Group B). Group A was selected to cover the most problematic period for rapid development of severe spine deformities, and Group B to give a broad representation of natural RS histories from an untreated adult population (≥18 years of age, median age 23 years). The basic data of the two groups in relation to the stage of disease are shown in Table 6.1.

II. Radiological and orthopaedic study
Of the 106 RS patients, 78 had had spine X-rays taken which were available to use for more systematic scoliosis analyses. The ages of these patients ranged from 1 to 34 years. X-ray films were measured retrospectively by two of us (E.S. and J.L.). There were a total of 149 sitting or standing X-rays. 37 patients had single exposures, while 41 had multiple observations, making progress and progress rate calculations possible. The follow-up time in the multiply observed patients was one

TABLE 6.1

Rett syndrome scoliosis study series: basic data

Age group	Distribution by stage of disease*		
	III	*IV-A*	*IV-B*
A (11–15 yrs)			
N	17	4	8
Median age	11½	12	11½
Age range	11–14	11–13	11–13
B (≥18 yrs)			
N	17	17	13
Median age	23	24	21
Age range	18–42	19–48	19–25

*See Chapter 2 for explanation of staging.

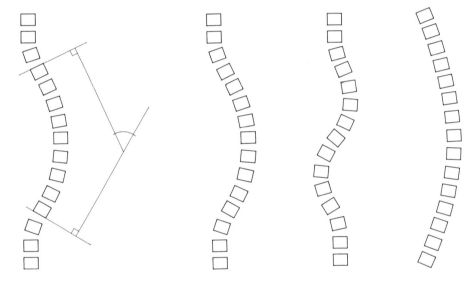

Fig. 6.1. Cobb's measurement of scoliosis angle. Lines are drawn perpendicular to a base line through the endplate of the neutral vertebra (where the angle changes direction).

Fig. 6.2. Curve types. *Left:* Normal pattern with one primary curve and two smaller compensatory curves above and below. The compensatory curves keep the spine in balance. *Centre:* Double primary curve—two opposite curves of the same magnitude (<5° difference) that balance each other. *Right:* C-shaped, so-called 'collapsing' type of curve.

to 14 years (mean 5 years 10 months). This series of patients is independent of that in study I.

In general we had access to anteroposterior spine radiographs, but in a few cases we had to measure chest X-rays. The Cobb angle (Fig. 6.1) was measured and the type of curvature (Fig. 6.2) was noted.

TABLE 6.2

Spine deformities in stage III patients

Age group	Scoliosis			High kyphosis	
	Insignificant or not noted	Obvious but moderate	Severe deformitive	Marked	Mild
A (N = 17)	5	12	0	1	5
B (N = 17)	5	11	1	7	4

TABLE 6.3

Spine deformities in stage IV-A patients

Age group	Scoliosis			Prominent high kyphosis
	Insignificant or not noted	Obvious but moderate	Severe deformitive	
A (N = 4)	0	3	1	0
B (N = 17)	0	6	11	0

TABLE 6.4

Spine deformities in stage IV-B patients

Age group	Scoliosis			Prominent high kyphosis
	Insignificant or not noted	Obvious but moderate	Severe deformitive	
A (N = 8)	0	1	7	0
B (N = 13)	0	1	12	0

Results

Study I. The neuropaediatric evaluation

TYPE OF SCOLIOSIS CURVE

Among those patients in whom a curvature was noted, the characteristic scoliosis was a double-curved thoracolumbar deformity, the convexity of the greater curve being right-sided in almost two-thirds, left-sided in around one third, and double primary in only a few.

BACK DEFORMITY RELATED TO STAGE OF DISEASE

When analysing the type and severity of spine deformity in relation to the various stages of disease (Tables 6.2–6.4) and the dominating neurology, the following pattern emerged.

Stage III. In group A (11–15 years), comprising 17 girls, the majority had a scoliosis which was mild (N=8) or moderate (N=2), and which did not seem to be clinically alarming. Three patients had either no spine deformity at all or only a questionable one. Two girls had a high, mainly cervical, kyphotic deformity, one of whom later had to be operated on. For these 15 patients the neurological picture was dominated by apraxia–ataxia. None had limb wasting, tendon reflexes were rarely exaggerated, and dystonic signs were absent. The remaining two patients had moderate but increasing and alarming scoliosis. One of them, aged 11 years, had asymmetrical dystonia in addition to her dominating apraxia–ataxia. The other, 12½ years old, had increasing lower motor neuron symptomatology with distal limb atrophy.

Among the 17 stage III women in group B (≥18 years), three had a very mild and clinically insignificant scoliosis, and nine, with a median age of 20½ years, had a spine deformity dominated more by a high cervicothoracic kyphosis than by a deforming scoliosis. With only two exceptions, the scoliosis was quite mild and considered stationary. One additional case had a short-curved low thoracic scoliosis considered secondary to a vertebral malformation. The remaining four women already had a deforming scoliosis (Fig. 6.3). Three of them had partial paralysis of the legs, sometimes with slight spasticity, in addition to the apraxia–ataxia. As in the younger age group, however, the majority of the stage III RS women had mainly apraxic–ataxic signs.

Stage IV-A. The back deformity was severe and/or threatening (one girl operated on at age 11) in the majority of stage IV-A patients in both age groups. The neurological findings in the younger patients (group A) were characterized by partial paralysis of trunk and limbs in addition to the basic apraxia–ataxia. In the adult group (group B) the findings were mixed, with partial limb paralysis, dystonia and/or spasticity, while the ataxic symptoms were in the main no longer obvious. In no stage IV-A patient was there a prominent high kyphotic deformity, in contrast to the pattern seen in the ambulant stage III group, particularly the adult cohort.

Stage IV-B. This stage comprises the most severely motor disabled and neurologically impaired RS females. All eight stage IV-B girls in group A had a history of early marked hypotonia, of lower limb weakness indicating early lower motor neuron impairment, and of successively increasing distal limb atrophy and abiotrophy, the latter affecting particularly the lower limbs. The spinal deformity in this group, with only one exception, was pronounced and of early onset. One of the girls had been operated on at 11 years of age, so far with excellent stabilization.

Of the 17 women in group B, 12 had very severe deformity and five had somewhat more moderate, yet clinically unacceptable, curvature. The underlying neurology seemed basically very similar to that in group A, though more difficult to appreciate in retrospect. Most of these older patients had never had a neurological examination at any time in their life. Thus, it was possible to determine only indirectly from parents and fragmentary records that a hypotonic partial paralysis

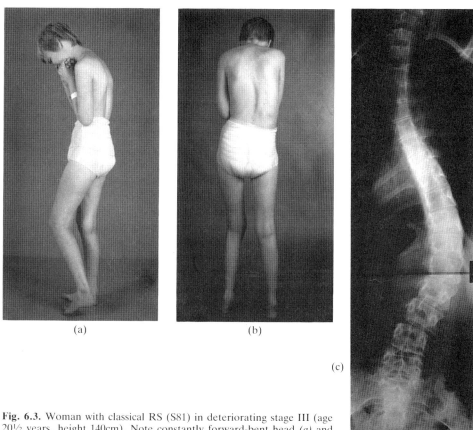

(a)　　　　　　　　　(b)

(c)

Fig. 6.3. Woman with classical RS (S81) in deteriorating stage III (age 20½ years, height 140cm). Note constantly forward-bent head *(a)* and upper back position *(b)*; *(c)* shows spine X-ray (frontal view).

had probably prevailed as an early manifestation. As adults, the women showed a complex mixture of signs. Sometimes there was a fixed rigid atrophic picture, impossible to elucidate even in its main components. This was the case particularly among those aged 25 years or older.

Study II. Radiological and orthopaedic results
For data analysis in this study the X-ray observations were divided into five age groups (0–5 years, 6–10 years, 11–15 years, 16–20 years, ≤21 years). As indicated in Table 6.5, there was a progression of curvature with age. The range of curvature was wide in all age groups, due to the mixture of cases in various stages of muscle weakness and neurological impairment. When the analysis was limited to first-time observations and to curvatures with a Cobb angle ≥10°, progression of scoliosis was still apparent, as seen in Table 6.6. The percentage of patients with radiologically confirmed scoliosis in the various age groups, as well as the proportion who had

65

TABLE 6.5

Total number of X-ray observations by age group

	Age group				
	0–5 yrs	6–10 yrs	11–15 yrs	16–20 yrs	≥21 yrs
Patients	16	29	32	18	16
Observations	20	39	50	23	17
Mean Cobb	15°	25°	38°	55°	48°
Median	14°	23°	33°	56°	37°
Range	0–38°	0–90°	0–84°	0–130°	0–108°

TABLE 6.6

First-time X-ray observations of scoliosis (Cobb ≥10°)

	Age group				
	0–5 yrs	6–10 yrs	11–15 yrs	16–20 yrs	≥21 yrs
N	11	14	20	7	11
Mean Cobb	22°	26°	30°	39°	60°
Range	10–38°	10–57°	10–81°	10–71°	10–108°

TABLE 6.7

Proportion of patients with scoliosis (Cobb ≥10°) at different ages

Age group (yrs)	0–5	6–10	11–15	16–20	≥21
Scoliosis (%)	~15	~30	~60	~65	~80

TABLE 6.8

Scoliosis curve progression rate in the 10 most severe cases, with mean age of patient

Progression rate (Cobb °/yr)	41	41	34	30	27	25	23	21	21	20
Age of patient (yrs)*		9	18	13	11	11	5	15	12	5	7

*Ages given are the mean age in the interval during which the progression occurred. The range of intervals was 6–21 months (mean 11 months).

scoliosis detected at first X-ray, are shown in Table 6.7. One third of 6- to 10-year-old girls had a scoliosis; among those ≥21 years the proportion increased to four fifths. The curve pattern analysis revealed that in 15 of the 78 patients (19 per cent) the curvature was of the C-shaped 'collapsing' type, while the remainder had the double curved pattern seen in idiopathic scoliosis.

The progress rate was calculated as the change in Cobb angle in degrees per year between two successive observations. The data for the ten most severe cases, related to the age when this progression happened, are given in Table 6.8. Neurologically these cases were characterized by early hypotonia, weakness and poor gross motor development. Some, in addition, had asymmetrical dystonic signs. In contrast, nine of the 41 patients with multiple observations did not show any progression of curvature. The mean observation time for this group was 3.8 years, and their mean age was 15.0 years. With one exception they were all ambulant stage III cases.

When correlating curve magnitude and progression with clinical staging of the disease the following was found. Of the total series, there were 13 patients (mean age 11 years), who showed a progression rate ⩾15°/year. Of these, six belonged to stage IV-A, four to stage IV-B and three to stage III. This finding should be compared with the group A data from the neuropaediatric study, where 17 of the 29 patients were in stage III, with four and eight respectively in stages IV-A and IV-B (Table 6.1). In the very young age group (0–5 years)—not yet represented in the neuropaediatric study—eight out of 16 patients had already developed a curvature >15°. They were all referred to clinically as severely motor impaired, often hypotonic at birth, and with early marked limb weakness. All but one have rapidly progressed to stage IV, mainly type IV-B.

Discussion

Scoliosis is a well recognized complication of many progressive neurological conditions (Hensinger and MacEwen 1976). The proportion of patients with different neuromuscular disorders having scoliosis varies from a few up to almost 100 per cent. The progression resembles the idiopathic type in that it usually occurs during the period of rapid growth (*i.e.* the second decade of life), although it tends to start earlier and to develop more quickly (Fisk and Bunch 1979). It also differs from the idiopathic type in that cessation of growth does not necessarily mean an arrest of curve progression. Neuromuscular scoliosis otherwise is known to develop in most cases the same curve pattern as that of idiopathic scoliosis (Fisk and Bunch 1979). However, patients with muscle paralysis or symmetrical muscle weakness tend to acquire a long C-shaped, so-called 'collapsing' type of curve.

As RS was unknown to the medical world until the mid-1980s, no systematic long-term follow-up study of the scoliosis so far exists. In trying to map the natural history of RS scoliosis from nationwide clinical material through various ages and stages we unfortunately have had to use two disparate series of data sources: one neuropaediatric, with scattered observations from clinical records and follow-up data, the other with unsystematically performed X-ray examinations, often with no or incomplete contemporary clinical records. Such a procedure has obvious weaknesses. Nevertheless, it has provided us with certain rough lines for understanding the appearance, the development and the background of the back deformities in RS girls of various types. The age groups chosen for study were centred on the growth spurt period between 11 and 15 years and on the final presentation in adulthood.

As the two series are disparate we found it necessary to present the data separately, under neuropaediatric and radiological–orthopaedic headings respectively, then combining the results to make our final conclusions.

Neuropaediatric aspects

The most important message has been that the patients at high risk of developing severe and rapidly progressing deformities, necessitating early supervision and surgical intervention, can be identified in early childhood. Analyses of the never-ambulant stage IV-B patients clearly indicates that such RS girls, with rare exceptions, are likely to have severe, early deformity. They will inevitably be wheelchair dependent, so to enable them to function and communicate as well as possible in adult life they must have the ability to sit reasonably well.

Today, untreated adult RS females in stage IV-B have a greatly reduced ability to sit due to their grotesque back deformities. As young girls they were characterized by marked hypotonia, partial lower limb paralysis and distal limb atrophy. We interpret the latter as being due to a complex dysfunction of both spinal (Oldfors *et al.* 1990) and central brain origin (Hagberg and Witt-Engerström 1986, Hagberg 1989, Witt-Engerström and Hagberg 1990). These extremely disabled patients contrasted with those in our series who had learned to walk and had remained mobile through the years, *i.e.* those in permanent stage III. The latter certainly all had prominent hand apraxia and gait dyspraxia with ataxic signs in addition, but with no, or only very mild, early distal limb weakness and atrophy. Thus there was a clear and early clinical distinction between the two extreme stages (III and IV-B), indicating that clinical differentiation was possible in the early preschool years.

A second message from our analysis is that basal ganglia dysfunction with limb dystonia is an ominous sign heralding future severe back deformity. Among our mobile stage III girls in group A, such cases had a bad back prognosis, and this was even more noticeable in the group B adults. Compared to the early manifestation of limb weakness, later appearing dystonic features tend to be increasingly asymmetrical. This is most dangerous, favouring a rapidly developing and malignant spinal curve deterioration.

A third finding was that just over half of all adult stage III RS women had a dominating high cervicothoracic kyphosis. This condition could be traced back to the group A (11–15 years) stage III group. With few exceptions, these girls did not develop a seriously progressive scoliosis. The kyphosis in the majority of cases was not incapacitating and, with only one exception, not clinically alarming. Thus, surgical intervention was usually unnecessary.

Radiological and orthopaedic aspects

Our data (Tables 6.5–6.7), showing that the proportion of RS patients developing scoliosis increased with age, correspond well to those of Bassett and Tolo (1990). Other investigators (Keret *et al.* 1988, Roberts and Conner 1988, Loder *et al.* 1989, Harrison and Webb 1990, Holm and King 1990) found between 42 and 83 per cent of RS patients with scoliosis, the differences mainly reflecting variations in age between the series.

The onset of scoliosis in RS occurs remarkably early, in general before that seen in other neuromuscular disorders. In our series 40 per cent of the curves had been discovered before the age of 11 (Table 6.7). Other investigators have given a mean age for onset of scoliosis of between 7 and 11 years (Keret *et al.* 1988, Loder *et al.* 1989, Harrison and Webb 1990, Holm and King 1990). Harrison and Webb found that 72 per cent of their patients had developed scoliosis before the age of 8. A rapid and severe progression also can no doubt occur very early, as noted in two of our patients by the age of 5 (Table 6.8).

Some patients in our study showed a very rapid curve progression, even faster than usually observed in traditional neuromuscular conditions (Hensinger and MacEwen 1976). Keret *et al.* (1988) also reported very rapidly progressive curves, particularly during the growth spurt. Contrary to these results, we found the rapid progression to be distributed over a wide range of ages, *i.e.* from 5 to 18 years. This accords with the observations of Holm and King (1990).

On the other hand, progression of curvature is not inevitable. No progression was seen in 17 per cent of our cases, and this may be a minimum figure as patients followed only by clinical observations were not included. Holm and King (1990) reported a progression rate of only 38 per cent, while other groups had up to 100 per cent (Keret *et al.* 1988, Loder *et al.* 1989).

Our series included mainly ordinary curve patterns with only a few of the collapsing type. This is in contrast to the series of Keret *et al.* (1988) and Guidera *et al.* (1991), the latter having exclusively collapsing types. Both these series, however, were small, with only eight and five RS patients respectively. In other studies (Hennessy and Haas 1988, Loder *et al.* 1989) normal curve patterns predominated.

Our data indicate a greater risk of rapid progression in patients in stage IV, and a markedly increased risk of rapid early curve development in young RS girls with marked hypotonia and muscular insufficiency. Naidu *et al.* (1986) also observed faster progress in non-ambulatory patients. Contrary to these findings, however, Holm and King (1990) reported that five out of eight patients with progression were ambulatory, while Harrison and Webb (1990) found early onset of scoliosis to correlate to stage III coupled to early puberty and increased height velocity.

From our X-ray data we cannot consider the problem of kyphosis because many of our radiograms did not include a lateral view. Data on kyphosis in RS have been given in several studies (Keret *et al.* 1988, Loder *et al.* 1989, Bassett and Tolo 1990, Guidera *et al.* 1991). While Keret *et al.* found no hyperkyphosis, Bassett and Tolo reported three patients who had undergone surgery for that deformity.

69

Certainly the problems connected to kyphosis seem less serious. Nevertheless, they should not be forgotten, particularly considering the relatively high frequency of such deformity in older stage III patients, as revealed in study I (see above).

Management of scoliosis in Rett syndrome
The problem of appropriate treatment for the RS scoliosis patient is still in great dispute. Many authors consider both brace treatment and surgery. However, there are still insufficient long-term experience and too few natural history data.

Bassett and Tolo (1990) recommend biannual clinical evaluation after the age of 5, and they believe that brace treatment may not alter the curve progression. They reported treatment of curves up to 56° Cobb angle, a curvature normally considered too great to respond to brace treatment even in ordinary idiopathic scoliosis. Our finding of scoliosis in certain children under 5 years old, with rapid progression in addition, indicates that clinical control only biannually could be hazardous. Our study points to the necessity of more frequently repeated clinical and radiological evaluations of children in early advanced neurological impairment. In fact, RS girls of any age, when noted to have early hypotonia and motor impairment, should be monitored meticulously for a developing scoliosis.

Harrison and Webb (1990) found that bracing beyond the age of 8 years had only a temporary effect on curve progression. They still recommended early brace treatment to postpone surgical intervention until the patient has developed a more mature skeletal structure. They also suggested brace treatment for patients in whom there is an imbalance or who have a curve exceeding 20 to 30° Cobb angle. For a scoliosis curve greater than 40° they recommended early fusion.

Our results point to the risk of progression for all children with early hypotonia and lower limb and trunk weakness who will either never reach a level of independent walking (stage IV-B) or rapidly deteriorate from an ambulant stage III to early wheelchair dependency (stage IV-A). For these patients, brace treatment, to have a chance to be effective, might have to start even before the Cobb angle reaches 20 to 30°. That might occur during the very early school years, mainly among those most severely motor disabled. For them, the only attainable goal could be a reasonable sitting posture for the rest of their lives. Certainly this is important, but other factors also have to be taken into consideration. In certain cases constant bracing is of doubtful benefit due to the complex asymmetrical neurological picture (Hagberg, personal observations). Moreover, bracing is sometimes badly tolerated by RS girls with their peculiar mood deviations. In some cases, we must accept that brace treatment does not work. In some situations one must either perform a primary fusion as soon as possible or accept that bracing may be more harmful to the patient than the loss of optimum sitting ability.

Conclusions
1. The scoliosis in RS is of a neurogenic type, of quite complex neurological origin, and develops earlier than idiopathic scoliosis.

2. The development of scoliosis is dependent more on complex neurological factors and stage of disease than on age.

3. Curve progression is usually more rapid than in idiopathic scoliosis and in most other types of neurogenic scoliosis in childhood, and occurs in a broader age span.

4. Early hypotonia, weakness and muscular insufficiency, and an early clinical referral to disease stages IV-A or IV-B are ominous factors.

5. Due to the complexity and to the large variation between cases, clinical follow-up of the scoliosis curve has to start early and be repeated regularly and frequently.

ACKNOWLEDGEMENTS

The study was supported by grants from W:6 Rett Research, 1991 and 1992.

REFERENCES

Bassett, G.S., Tolo, V.T. (1990) 'The incidence and natural history of scoliosis in Rett syndrome.' *Developmental Medicine and Child Neurology*, **32**, 963–966.

Fisk, J.R., Bunch, W.H. (1979) 'Scoliosis in neuromuscular disease.' *Orthopedic Clinics of North America*, **10**, 863–875.

Guidera, K.J., Borrelli, J., Raney, E., Thompson-Rangel, T., Ogden, J.A. (1991) 'Orthopaedic manifestations of Rett syndrome.' *Journal of Pediatric Orthopaedics*, **11**, 204–208.

Hagberg, B. (1989) 'Rett syndrome: clinical pecularities, diagnostic approach and possible cause.' *Pediatric Neurology*, **5**, 75–83.

—— Witt-Engerström, I. (1986) 'Rett syndrome: a suggested staging system for describing impairment profile with increasing age towards adolescence.' *American Journal of Medical Genetics*, **24** (Suppl. 1), 47–59.

—— Aicardi, J., Dias, K., Ramos, O. (1983) 'A progressive syndrome of autism, dementia, ataxia, and loss of purposeful hand use in girls: Rett syndrome: report of 35 cases.' *Annals of Neurology*, **14**, 471–479.

Harrison, D.J., Webb, P.J. (1990) 'Scoliosis in the Rett syndrome: natural history and treatment.' *Brain and Development*, **12**, 154–156.

Hennessy, M.J., Haas, R.H. (1988) 'The orthopedic management of Rett syndrome.' *Journal of Child Neurology*, **3** (Suppl.), S43–S47.

Hensinger, R.N., MacEwen, G.D. (1976) 'Spinal deformity associated with heritable neurological conditions: spinal muscular atrophy, Friedreich's ataxia, familial dysautonomia, and Charcot-Marie-Tooth disease.' *Journal of Bone and Joint Surgery*, **58A**, 13–24.

Holm, V.A., King, H.A. (1990) 'Scoliosis in the Rett syndrome.' *Brain and Development*, **12**, 151–153.

Keret, D., Bassett, G.S., Bunnell, W.P., Marks, H.G. (1988) 'Scoliosis in Rett syndrome.' *Journal of Pediatric Orthopaedics*, **8**, 138–142.

Loder, R.T., Lee, C.L., Richards, B.S. (1989) 'Orthopaedic aspects of Rett syndrome: a multicenter review.' *Journal of Pediatric Orthopaedics*, **9**, 557–562.

Naidu, S., Murphy, M., Moser, H.W., Rett, A. (1986) 'Rett syndrome—Natural history in 70 cases. *American Journal of Medical Genetics*, **24** (Suppl. 1), 61–72.

Oldfors, A., Hagberg, B., Nordgren, H., Sourander, P., Witt-Engerström, I. (1988) 'Rett syndrome: spinal cord neuropathology.' *Pediatric Neurology*, **4**, 172–174.

Roberts, A.P., Conner, A.N. (1988) 'Orthopaedic aspects of Rett's syndrome; brief report.' *Journal of Bone and Joint Surgery*, **70B**, 674.

Witt Engerström, I. (1990) 'Rett syndrome in Sweden. Neurodevelopment – Disability – Pathophysiology.' *Acta Paediatrica Scandinavica*, Suppl. 369.

—— Hagberg, B. (1990) 'The Rett syndrome: gross motor disability and neural impairment in adults.' *Brain and Development*, **12**, 23–26.

7
NEUROPHYSIOLOGICAL DIAGNOSIS

Gaby Bader and Ingrid Hagne

The electroencephalogram (EEG) has been widely used in the diagnosis of Rett syndrome, especially as epilepsy is a component of the clinical picture in most patients. The early report by Hagberg *et al.* (1983), based on data from 35 French, Portuguese and Swedish patients aged 2 to 22 years, stressed the presence of bilaterally synchronous paroxysmal slow spike–wave complexes in sleep records and a successively flattening record when awake. In the following years several EEG studies of RS patients were published, including some based on larger samples (Niedermeyer *et al.* 1986, Verma *et al.* 1986, Glaze *et al.* 1987, Robb *et al.* 1989). In some reports the EEG findings were correlated to the clinical stages of the disease, as defined by Hagberg and Witt-Engerström (1986) and detailed in Chapter 2. 127 EEG recordings of 30 Swedish patients were studied in detail with special reference to the developmental aspects of the EEG (Hagne *et al.* 1989). As is obvious from the clinical picture of RS, not only the brain but also the spinal cord is involved in the disease. Thus, in studying the disorder other neurophysiological methods in addition to EEG have been applied, including somatosensory and brainstem evoked potentials, conduction velocity of peripheral nerves and electromyography (EMG).

EEG findings

During *stage I* the EEG is usually normal, sometimes slightly slow. From around age 2 to 3 years, in clinical *stage II*, epileptic seizures are characteristic. The typical corresponding EEG finding, which sometimes precedes the start of clinical seizures, is focal spikes in central, often centroparietal (parasagittal) leads (Verma *et al.* 1986, Robertson *et al.* 1988, Hagne *et al.* 1989, Robb *et al.* 1989, Aldrich *et al.* 1990, Niedermeyer and Naidu 1990). The spikes are seen in one or both hemispheres, synchronously or independently, in the waking EEG, but most consistently in sleep records. During sleep the focal spike activity is often almost continuous (Fig. 7.1). The central spikes were facilitated in some patients by contralateral tactile stimulation (Robb *et al.* 1989) and in certain cases attenuated by passive finger movements (Niedermeyer and Naidu 1990). In different reports the incidence of parasagittal spikes in stage II varies around 60 to 70 per cent, but in our expereince is higher. During the course of stage II, however, several other epileptic patterns are seen, such as multifocal spikes and bilaterally synchronous bursts of irregular spike and slow wave discharges. Although characteristic of stage II, central spikes sometimes persist in stage III.

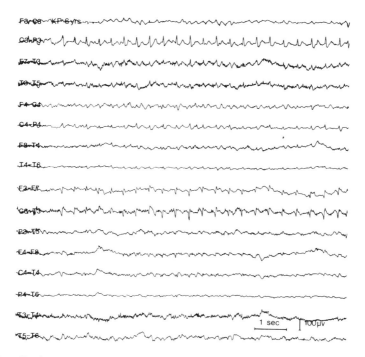

Fig. 7.1. Continuous spike activity in left central leads in 6-year-old girl with stage II RS.

Epileptic discharges are, however, less frequent in *stage III*, as are clinical seizures. In this clinically rather uneventful period some rare EEG patterns develop, mainly in sleep recordings. The normal EEG morphology of sleep disappears and in many cases is replaced by intermittent bursts of irregular delta waves, appearing against a rather flat background (Fig. 7.2*a*). A less pronounced periodic pattern can be seen in drowsiness, consisting of discrete theta episodes. The intermittent delta burst pattern is, as pointed out by Trauner and Haas (1987), strikingly similar to that seen in subacute sclerosing panencephalitis (SSPE) (Fig. 7.2*b*). In the study by Hagne *et al.* (1989), this pattern was present throughout the sleep recording, with delta episodes of 1 to 1.5s duration. Their frequency varied between 12 and 15 complexes per minute, with a tendency toward longer intervals in deep sleep. The amplitudes of the episodes increased with sleep depth, concomitantly with flattening of the intervals. No clinical correlates of the bursts were observed. Nine out of 15 girls observed in stage III displayed an intermittent EEG sleep pattern. This pattern persisted in four of 12 girls examined in stage IV.

In *stage IV*, further abnormal patterns may be found, mostly of an epileptic character although seizures are generally not a prominent feature of the clinical picture in this stage. In the study by Hagne *et al.* (1989) four of 12 patients showed a pattern of status epilepticus in waking and sleep records, with around 1Hz continuous rhythmic bilaterally synchronous and generalized spikes (Fig. 7.3). The

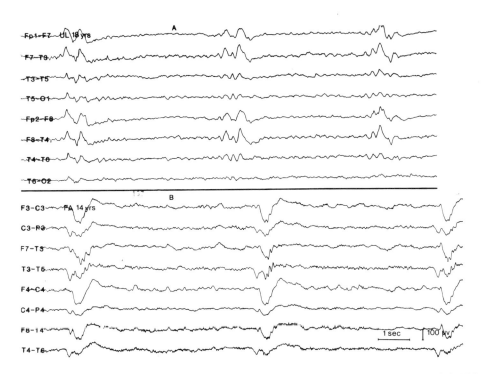

Fig. 7.2. (A) Pseudoperiodic delta episodes during sleep in 18-year-old girl with stage III RS. (B) EEG of 14-year-old girl with subacute sclerosing panencephalitis.

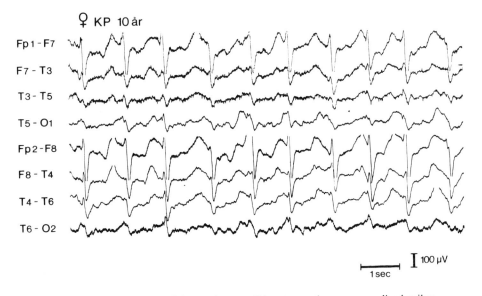

Fig. 7.3. Same patient as in Figure 7.1, now in stage IV: note continuous generalized spikes.

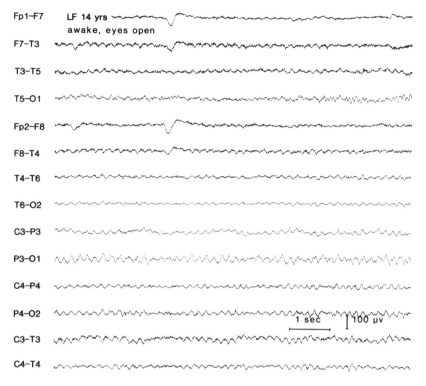

Fig. 7.4. Generalized monorhythmic non-reactive 5Hz activity in 14-year-old girl with stage IV RS.

patients had only occasional seizures. We tried in one patient to control the electrographic status with intravenous infusion of barbiturate and diazepam, but without improvement of either the EEG pattern or clinical state. Another pattern, described by Niedermeyer *et al.* (1986), consists of a monorhythmic generalized 3 to 5Hz activity in awake and drowsy states (Fig. 7.4). This rhythm is not reactive to stimuli. We saw that pattern in three out of 12 stage IV patients and in two out of 16 stage III patients.

Beside the patterns described, the progress of the disease is also reflected as *slowing of the alpha-rhythm*, which is often completely suppressed, in some patients replaced by the aforementioned non-reactive slow rhythm.

Episodes of *hyperventilation alternating with apnoeic periods* and *stereotypic hand movements* are characteristic behavioural deviations in Rett patients. Neither the hand movements nor the apnoea have been shown to correlate with paroxysmal events in the EEG or with the intermittent patterns of drowsiness and sleep.

Disturbances of the awake–sleep rhythm of Rett patients are quite often reported by their parents. As mentioned, in conventional daytime sleep recordings the normal morphology of sleep, including sleep spindles and vertex sharp waves, is disturbed, often being absent in stages III and IV. Some *polygraphic* EEG studies of all night sleep in RS have been performed. Segawa and Nomura (1990) found disturbances of sleep stages which they interpreted as suggestive of a dysfunction of the monoamine metabolism of midbrain and brainstem neurons. Aldrich *et al.* (1990) focused on the incidence of spike activity. They found spikes most frequent in non-REM sleep, increasing during the second half of the night. Significantly more total sleep in Rett patients than in age-matched controls was reported by Piazza *et al.* (1990). The sleep also showed abnormal distribution over night and day with diminished night sleep and increased daytime sleep.

Thus, in summary, the EEG in RS shows a characteristic staged progression which corresponds with the clinical stages:

- Stage I: normal EEG
- Stage II: central spikes, followed by other epileptic patterns, *i.e.* multifocal or bilaterally synchronous spikes and slow waves
- Stage III: intermittent delta and theta bursts with flat intervals, or monorhythmic slow activity
- Stage IV: continuous generalized rhythmic spikes.

In contrast to the grossly abnormal patterns described, single patients may in stage IV exhibit a normal, low voltage record. The progress of the EEG abnormality is usually slow but, especially in the later stages of RS, the pattern varies considerably between individuals. Thus we observed one girl pass within a few years through EEG stages II to IV, concomitantly with a rapid clinical deterioration.

The appearance in stages III and IV of periodic EEG patterns, otherwise seen almost exclusively in slow virus encephalitides, SSPE and, in stage IV, Creutzfeldt–Jakob disease, is hard to understand, as the underlying patho-anatomical features are quite different.

For clinical diagnostic purposes the EEG is useful, especially in stage II where the clinical differential diagnosis between RS and other progressive brain diseases such as infantile ceroid lipofuscinosis and Angelman syndrome is often difficult.

Peripheral nerve and EMG studies
A few neurophysiological investigations of peripheral nerve and muscle have been published. Jellinger *et al.* (1990) studied four girls with RS in stages II and III. They found motor nerve conduction velocities (NCVs) and distal latencies within normal values in the upper limbs, but distal latencies for the peroneal nerve were increased in two girls and compound muscle action potential was abnormal in one. The authors concluded that the lower motor neuron involvement may be due to mild distal axonopathy of unknown origin rather than to primary spinal cord involvement. In a study of 13 RS girls aged 2 to 16 years, of whom 10 had NCV measurements taken, Espinar-Sierra *et al.* (1990) found an increased distal motor latency in the peroneal nerve in only one, whereas six had an abnormal EMG, indicating peripheral nerve damage. In two girls spontaneous denervation activity was noted.

The Swedish group of Bader *et al.* (1989) studied motor and sensory NCVs in 13 patients with RS (one in stage III, 12 in stage IV). They found a slightly lowered motor NCV in the lower limb in four girls, otherwise normal NCVs and normal distal latencies. In some patients the amplitude of the compound muscle action potential was low, indicating a loss of neurons. EMG in six patients was essentially normal, but in two of them slight changes of neurogenic type were found. (EMG investigation, however, is difficult to perform adequately in people with mental and physical disabilities because they are unable to cooperate.)

Thus, the examination of peripheral nerve and muscle in RS has shown occasional and mostly slight signs of peripheral nerve damage but no signs of major motor peripheral neuropathy even in advanced stages of RS.

Somatosensory evoked responses (SERs)

SERs are conducted by peripheral nerves through the spinal cord and the brainstem, the thalamus and the thalamocortical radiation to the cerebral cortex. Pathology on any of these levels can delay the transmission of impulses. White matter disease should affect these potentials.

Kálmánchey (1990) found all modalities of evoked responses normal in a group of five children aged 18 months to 4½ years. She concluded that RS is a predominantly grey matter disease. Verma *et al.* (1987) in a study of young RS girls came to the same conclusion.

The Bader *et al.* (1989) study included stimulation of the median nerves at the wrist. Evoked potentials were monitored at Erb's point, at the sixth cervical vertebral body and on the scalp overlying the contralateral somatosensory area. Cortical SER's were recorded by stimulation of the posterior tibial nerves. In eight of the 13 subjects recordings were also made in the popliteal fossa and along the spinal cord. All patients investigated showed some abnormality of SER, asymmetry, delayed latency and/or a prolonged conduction time. None showed a delayed response at Erb's point, but most had delayed response at the cervical level in comparison to height-matched controls. The finding of a prolonged conduction time from brachial plexus to the cervical spine may indicate slowing of conduction in the sensory roots. Deformity of the spine may, however, lead to slowing due to medullary compression; it can also interfere with accurate measurement of height, leading to erronous interpretation of the height-dependent conduction time between Erb's point and the cervical spine. The RS patients, with a deformed spine (age range 10–22 years; height range 116–152cm), were initially compared to teenage/young adult controls with a normal spine (*i.e.* roughly matched for age but not height): no significant difference was found between the two groups. However, when compared to a younger (<13 years), height-matched control group, the mean conduction time was shown to be increased in the patients.

The central conduction time (CCT), which is independent of height, was often increased. The CCT is affected by selective loss of fibres in central pathways.

When lower limb SERs were investigated, delayed cortical responses were found in all patients. On segmental measurements, the conduction time between the popliteal fossa and the spine was found to be normal, but the CCT between spinal and cortical responses was increased, indicating that the delay occurred proximal to the spinal recordings.

SER findings thus gave evidence of dysfunction of the spinal medulla and the spinothalamic tract.

Motor evoked potentials

The excitability of corticospinal neurons was investigated by Eyre *et al*. (1990). Electromagnetic stimulation of the motor cortex and cervical motor roots was used to evoke motor action potentials in muscles of the upper limb. While cervical motor root stimulation resulted in responses of normal latency and duration, motor cortex stimulation evoked responses with a prolonged duration. The authors concluded that the corticospinal pathway was intact and suggested a disordered synaptic control of the motor cortex and/or the spinal motor neuron.

Visual evoked responses (VERs)

Only flash VERs can be used in uncooperative patients because that method is independent of attention or alertness. Kálmánchey (1990) found normal flash VERs in five RS patients. Bader *et al*. (1989) found a slightly increased latency of the mean first positive wave for their patient group (p<0.05) as compared to a normal control group. It was not possible to determine whether the delay of the responses was due to slowed conduction in the optic tract, or to cortical or subcortical lesions.

Auditory evoked responses

The Swedish patient group showed variable abnormalities along the auditory pathways (Bader *et al*. 1989). Delayed latency and/or prolonged conduction time for the auditory brainstem evoked response and the middle late response suggested lesions at the brainstem and at a higher level. The presence of the sometimes delayed auditory cortical response and its normal scalp distribution led to the conclusion that these patients retain higher hearing functions.

Conclusion

Neurophysiological investigations have contributed to the understanding of the pathophysiology of RS. EEG is useful in the diagnosis and differential diagnosis from clinical stage II onwards. At that time focal parasagittal spikes suggest a primarily cortical involvement. The abnormal EEG patterns seen in advanced stages of RS, however, apparently have a subcortical origin. Sensory evoked potentials in advanced RS indicate involvement of subcortical and spinal white matter structures. Investigations of peripheral nerves and muscles, on the other hand, give more doubtful results. NCVs are essentially normal, though studies in individual patients have shown some evidence of a peripheral neuropathy.

REFERENCES

Aldrich, M.S., Garofalo, E.A., Drury, I. (1990) 'Epileptiform abnormalities during sleep in Rett syndrome.' *Electroencephalography and Clinical Neurophysiology*, **75**, 365–370.

Bader, G.G., Witt-Engerström, I., Hagberg, B. (1989) 'Neurophysiological findings in the Rett syndrome. I: EMG, conduction velocity, EEG and somatosensory-evoked potential studies.' *Brain and Development*, **11**, 102–109.

Espinar-Sierra, J., Toledano, M.A., Franco, C., Campos-Castello, J., Gonzales-Hidalgo, M., Oliete, F., Garcia-Nart, M. (1990) 'Rett's syndrome: a neurophysiological study.' *Neurophysiologie Clinique*, **20**, 35–42.

Eyre, J.A., Kerr, A.M., Miller, S., O'Sullivan, M., Ramesh, V. (1990) 'Neurophysiological observations on corticospinal projections to the upper limb in subjects with Rett syndrome.' *Journal of Neurology, Neurosurgery and Psychiatry*, **53**, 874–879.

Glaze, D.G., Frost, J.D., Zoghbi, H.Y., Percy, A.K. (1987) 'Rett's syndrome. Correlation of electroencephalographic characteristics with clinical staging.' *Archives of Neurology*, **44**, 1053–1056.

Hagberg, B., Witt-Engerström, I. (1986) 'Rett syndrome: a suggested staging system for describing impairment profile with increasing age towards adolescence.' *American Journal of Medical Genetics*, **24**, (Suppl. 1), 47–59.

—— Aicardi, J., Dias, K., Ramos, O. (1983) 'A progressive syndrome of autism, dementia, ataxia and loss of purposeful hand use in girls: Rett's syndrome: Report of 35 cases.' *Annals of Neurology*, **14**, 471–479.

Hagne, I., Witt-Engerström, I., Hagberg, B. (1989) 'EEG development in Rett syndrome. A study of 30 cases.' *Electroencephalography and Clinical Neurophysiology*, **72**, 1–6.

Jellinger, K., Grisold, W., Armstrong, D., Rett, A. (1990) 'Peripheral nerve involvement in the Rett syndrome.' *Brain and Development*, **12**, 109–114.

Kálmánchey, R. (1990) 'Evoked potentials in the Rett syndrome.' *Brain and Development*, **12**, 73–76.

Niedermeyer, E., Naidu, S. (1990) 'Further EEG observations in children with the Rett syndrome.' *Brain and Development*, **12**, 53–54.

—— Rett, A., Renner, H., Murphy, M., Naidu, S. (1986) 'Rett syndrome and the electroencephalogram.' *American Journal of Medical Genetics*, **24** (Suppl. 1), 195–199.

Piazza, C., Fisher, W., Kiesewetter, K., Bowman, L., Moser, H. (1990) 'Aberrant sleep patterns in children with the Rett syndrome.' *Brain and Development*, **12**, 488–493.

Robb, S.A., Harden, A., Boyd, S.G. (1989) 'Rett syndrome: an EEG study in 52 girls.' *Neuropediatrics*, **20**, 192–195.

Robertson, R., Langill, L., Wong, P.K.H., Ho, H.H. (1988) 'Rett syndrome: EEG presentation.' *Electroencephalography and Clinical Neurophysiology*, **70**, 388–395.

Segawa, M., Nomura, Y. (1990) 'The pathophysiology of the Rett syndrome from the standpoint of polysomnography.' *Brain and Development*, **12**, 55–60.

Trauner, D.A., Haas, R.H. (1987) 'Electroencephalographic abnormalities in Rett's syndrome.' *Pediatric Neurology*, **3**, 331–334.

Verma, N.P., Chhedra, R.L., Nigro, M.A., Hart, Z.H. (1986) 'Electrocencephalographic findings in Rett syndrome.' *Electroencephalography and Clinical Neurophysiology*, **64**, 394–401.

—— Nigro, M.A., Hart, Z.H. (1987) 'Rett Syndrome—a gray matter disease? Electrophysiologic evidence.' *Electroencephalography and Clinical Neurophysiology*, **67**, 327–329.

8

REGIONAL CEREBRAL BLOOD FLOW: SPECT AS A TOOL FOR LOCALIZATION OF BRAIN DYSFUNCTION

Paul Uvebrant, Jan Bjure, Rune Sixt, Ingegerd Witt Engerström and Bengt Hagberg

Introduction

Surprisingly few neuroanatomical correlates of Rett syndrome have been found despite its functionally devastating effect. The comparatively subtle findings from magnetic resonance imaging (MRI) and computed tomography (CT) have been a small brain with some cortical atrophy (Krägeloh-Mann *et al.* 1989, Suzuki *et al.* 1989, Nihei and Naitoh 1990). Neuropathology has mainly revealed diffuse brain growth arrest with some atrophy (Jellinger and Seitelberger 1986, Nomura and Segawa 1986, Riederer *et al.* 1986, Jellinger *et al.* 1988, Oldfors *et al.* 1990).

Complementary techniques are needed to widen knowledge of early progressive cerebral pathophysiology. The measurement of regional cerebral blood flow (rCBF) has provided new and important information on a variety of dysfunctional states in the CNS, such as epilepsy (*Lancet* 1989), dementia (Neary *et al.* 1987, Zilbovicius *et al.* 1989), autism (Gaffney *et al.* 1989) and language disorders (Denays *et al.* 1989), all with sparse and often non-specific findings when investigated by CT/MRI.

The application of rCBF measurement techniques such as single photon emission computed tomography (SPECT) on girls with RS has indicated a preserved immature pattern of frontal lobe hypoperfusion in older patients (Nielsen *et al.* 1990). The purpose of the study reported here was to obtain additional information by the use of the recently introduced radiopharmaceutical HM-PAO (Ceretec®). The study was centred on young RS girls in an effort to discover early involved and likely pathophysiologically relevant areas of dysfunction, rather than mapping late and potentially secondary lesions.

Patients

The series is presented in Table 8.1. Ten girls with characteristic RS phenotypes were studied (median age 3½ years). Only three were over 4 years old at examination (9, 13 and 24 years respectively). Of the seven very young RS girls, all had by April 1992 passed the age limit for inclusion in the Swedish RS series (see Chapter 3). The criteria and stage of disease have been classified according to the Swedish system detailed in Chapter 2. Ten age-matched patients with other

TABLE 8.1

TABLE 8.1

Ages and clinical characteristics of RS study group, and ages of controls

Subject*	Age at investigation (yrs)	Age at June 1992 (yrs)	Rett stage at examination	Epilepsy	Age of controls (yrs)
S105	1½	3¾	II/III	No	¾
S114	1¾	3	II	Yes	1
S99	2½	5	III	No	2
S95	3¼	6	III/IV	No	3¾
S110	3¼	4½	III/IV	No	3½
S93	3½	6	III	Yes	4
S80	4	6¾	III/IV	Yes	7
S74	9¼	11	III	Yes	7½
S19	13½	16½	IV	Yes	12¾
S11	24¼	26½	IV	Yes	19¾

*Case numbers refer to Swedish Rett syndrome series detailed in Chapter 3.

neurological disorders served as controls, of whom six were younger than 4 years and seven were girls.

Method

An intravenous cannula was inserted 30 minutes before the injection of 10MBq Tc-99m HM-PAO per kg body weight. The child was examined in the supine position under general anaesthesia and with the head fixed. Tomography was performed with a GE 400 AT gamma camera fitted with a high resolution collimator using 64 projections (128*128 matrix; 30s per frame) and an elliptical orbit. Transaxial, coronal and sagittal slices (3mm thick) were reconstructed using prefiltering (Hanning $0.88cm^{-1}$) and ramp back projection. Irregular regions of interest were used to compare the uptake in various areas on a mean count/pixel basis. To ascertain good image quality a new uniformity correction map was acquired on the same day as the investigation and energy correction maps once a month. The system's centre of rotation was checked regularly.

Statistical analysis

A two-sided paired t-test was used for testing differences in the rCBF between RS patients and controls. A *p* value ≤0.05 was considered statistically significant. The 95 per cent confidence intervals of differences were calculated.

Results

Table 8.2 shows the rCBF ratios of the left and right hemisphere or lobe in RS patients and controls, as well as ratios of the lobes or midbrain regions and the cerebellum or whole hemisphere. Significantly reduced mean perfusion ratios in RS patients as compared with controls were found in the basal central parts of the brain, corresponding to the midbrain and upper brainstem, and the cerebellum

TABLE 8.2
Comparison of regional cerebral blood flow ratios in RS study group and controls

Region	RS subjects (N = 10)	Controls (N = 10)	p	95% confidence interval of difference
Hemispheres				
Left/right	1.00	1.03	*ns*	−0.060 to 0.002
Frontal lobes				
Left/right	0.99	1.01	<0.05	−0.031 to −0.001
Left/cerebellum	0.90	0.93	*ns*	−0.082 to 0.008
Right/cerebellum	0.90	0.93	*ns*	−0.068 to 0.016
Frontal/hemispheres	0.23	0.29	<0.001	−0.079 to −0.035
Temporal lobes				
Left/right	0.98	0.98	*ns*	−0.040 to 0.036
Left/cerebellum	0.84	0.88	<0.05	−0.083 to −0.001
Right/cerebellum	0.87	0.91	*ns*	−0.102 to 0.020
Midbrain/cerebellum	0.72	0.84	<0.001	−0.167 to −0.077

(14%, p<0.001); in the ratio of the frontal lobes and the hemispheres (21%; p<0.001); in the ratios of the left and right frontal lobes (p<0.05), and in that of the left temporal lobe and the cerebellum (p<0.05).

A general hemisphere asymmetry was not seen. Fig. 8.1*a* illustrates the hypoperfused areas in the midbrain/brainstem and frontal lobes. Figs. 8.1*b* and 8.1*c* show the normal perfusion pattern in an age-matched control and the immature low frontal lobe perfusion in a 7-week-old boy.

Discussion

No overall valid asymmetry between the left and right hemispheres in *regional cerebral perfusion* was found in our RS series. This is at variance with the findings of Nielsen *et al.* (1990), who demonstrated a shift to left hemisphere blood flow dominance in their (on average older) RS patients. The only significant left/right difference in the present study was a left frontotemporal hypoperfusion. This might indicate an early appearing left asymmetrical frontotemporal dysfunction in RS.

Our finding of *frontal lobe hypoperfusion* supported the 'immature' frontal lobe hypoperfusion pattern reported by Nielsen *et al.* (1990) in RS patients. Frontal lobe involvement has also been indicated in studies using MRI (Nihei and Naitoh 1990) and positron emission tomography (PET) (Yoshikawa *et al.* 1991). PET studies have otherwise been contradictory (Harris *et al.* 1986, Wagner 1986, Naidu *et al.* 1988).

The finding of *hypoperfusion in midbrain/brainstem* areas, as revealed by this study, has not been reported earlier. The spatial resolution of the SPECT technique of about 15mm did not allow for further delineation of involved

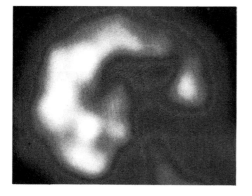

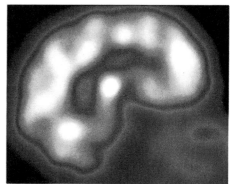

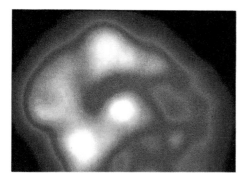

Fig. 8.1. SPECT scans revealing regional cerebral blood flow. *Top left:* 2½-year-old girl with RS: sagittal view of hypoperfusion in midbrain/upper brainstem area and frontal lobes. *Top right:* 1½-year-old control. *Opposite:* 7-week-old control: note immature low blood flow in frontal lobes and preserved high flow in midbrain/upper brainstem area.

structures. It may even be that the reduced perfusion in the midbrain and upper brainstem region represents not only reduced perfusion of brain tissue, but also local nerve cell loss in these areas as indicated by MRI findings of widening of the prepontine cistern and narrowing of the brainstem (Suzuki *et al.* 1989, Nihei and Naitoh 1990). The relevance of pathology in the midbrain was supported by the finding of a tumour in the corresponding area in another RS patient (a 4-year old girl not included in the present series—Fig 8.2). In this girl the brain lesion may represent the aetiology of the RS.

Midbrain and brainstem dysfunction in RS has been demonstrated by auditory brainstem evoked response measurements (see Chapter 7) and is also indicated by clinical symptoms such as breathing irregularities and sleep disturbances (Glaze *et. al.* 1987, Segawa and Nomura 1990). Even autism, a prominent feature in RS stage II, has been associated with midbrain and brainstem dysfunction (Hoshino *et al.* 1984, Steffenburg 1991). The pathophysiological mechanisms by which the brainstem/midbrain impairment causes or contributes to the development of RS are still obscure. Nomura *et al.* (1987) suggested a very early deficiency of the monoaminergic systems leading to serious abnormality in higher centres during development. It could be hypothesized that the 'immature' frontal lobe hypo-

83

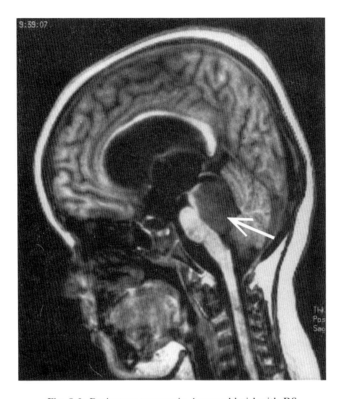

Fig. 8.2. Brainstem tumour in 4-year-old girl with RS.

perfusion pattern in RS might be the effect of early deficiencies in transmitter, brain growth and maturational systems, beginning in midbrain/brainstem structures. This possibility, repeatedly emphasized by the Segawa team (Nomura *et al.* 1987, Segawa and Nomura 1990) has been further strengthened through data reported at the 1990 Tokyo RS symposium (Segawa 1992).

Conclusions
In comparison with controls, Rett patients have a significant and early appearing hypoperfusion in the area of the midbrain and upper brainstem as well as the frontal lobes. Whether this pathology has developed in parallel in the two different brain localities, or if one of them has a leading, primary importance, is still an open question.

ACKNOWLEDGEMENTS

The study was supported by grants from the following foundations: Vera and Hans Albrechtson, W:6 Rett Research, Frimurare-Barnhusdirektionen, Göteborg Medical Society, M. and P. Molin, and Petter Silfverskiöld.

REFERENCES

Denays, R., Tondeur, M., Foulon, M., Verstraeten, F., Ham, H., Piepsz, A., Noel, P. (1989) 'Regional brain blood flow in congenital dysphasia: studies with technetium-99m-HMPAO SPECT.' *Journal of Nuclear Medicine*, **30**, 1825–1829.

Gaffney, G.R., Kuperman, S., Tsai, L.Y., Minchin, S. (1989) 'Forebrain structures in infantile autism.' *Journal of the American Academy of Child and Adolescent Psychiatry*, **28**, 534–537.

Glaze, D.G., Frost, J.D., Zoghbi, H.Y., Percy, A.K. (1987) 'Rett's syndrome: characterization of respiratory patterns and sleep.' *Annals of Neurology*, **21**, 377–382.

Harris, J.C., Wong, D.F., Wagner, H.N., Rett, A., Naidu, S., Dannals, R.F., Links, J.M., Batshaw, M.L., Moser, H.W. (1986) 'Positron emission tomographic study of D2 dopamine receptor binding CSF biogenic amine metabolites in Rett syndrome.' *American Journal of Medical Genetics*, **24** (Suppl. 1), 201–210.

Hoshino, Y., Manome, T., Kaneko, M., Yashima, Y., Kumashiro, H. (1984) 'Computed tomography of the brain in children with early infantile autism.' *Folia Psychiatrica Neurologica Japonica*, **38**, 33–43.

Jellinger, K., Seitelberger, F. (1986) 'Neuropathology of Rett syndrome.' *American Journal of Medical Genetics*, **24** (Suppl. 1), 259–288.

—— Armstrong, D., Zoghbi, H.Y., Percy, A.K. (1988) 'Neuropathology of Rett syndrome.' *Acta Neuropathologica*, **76**, 142–158.

Krägeloh-Mann, I., Schroth, G., Niemann, G., Michaelis, R. (1989) 'The Rett syndrome: magnetic resonance imaging and clinical findings in four girls.' *Brain and Development*, **11**, 175–178.

Lancet (1989) 'SPECT and PET in epilepsy.' *Lancet*, **i**, 135–137. (*Editorial.*)

Naidu, S., Wong, D.F., Sanche Roa, P., Dillemagne, V., Yaster, M., Dannals, R.F., Links, J., Wilson, A., Raveri, H., Harris, J., *et al.* (1988) 'Rett syndrome: positron emission tomography, metabolic–clinical correlates.' *Annals of Neurology*, **24**, 305. *(Abstract.)*

Neary, D., Snowden, J.S., Shields, R.A., Burjan, B., Northen, N., MacDermott, M.C., Prescott, H.J., Testa, N.J. (1987) 'Single photon emission tomography using ^{99m}Tc-HM-PAO in the investigation of dementia'. *Journal of Neurology, Neurosurgery and Psychiatry*, **50**, 1101–1109.

Nielsen, J.B., Friberg, L., Lou, H., Lassen, N.A., Sam, I.L. (1990) 'Immature pattern of brain activity in Rett syndrome.' *Archives of Neurology*, **47**, 982–986.

Nihei, K., Naitoh, H. (1990) 'Cranial computed tomographic and magnetic resonance imaging studies in the Rett syndrome.' *Brain and Development*, **12**, 101–105.

Nomura, Y., Segawa, M. (1986) 'Anatomy of Rett syndrome.' *American Journal of Medical Genetics*, **24**, (Suppl. 1), 289–303.

—— Honda, K., Segawa, M. (1987) 'Pathophysiology of Rett syndrome.' *Brain and Development*, **9**, 506–513.

Oldfors, A., Sourander, P., Armstrong, D.L., Percy, A.K., Witt Engerström, I., Hagberg, B.A. (1990) 'Rett syndrome: cerebellar pathology.' *Pediatric Neurology*, **6**, 310–314.

Riederer, P., Weiser, M., Wichart, I., Schmidt, B., Killian, W., Rett, A. (1986) 'Preliminary brain autopsy findings in progredient Rett syndrome.' *American Journal of Medical Genetics*, **24** (Suppl. 1), 305–315.

Segawa, M. (1992) 'Possible lesions of the Rett syndrome: opinions of contributors.' *Brain and Development*, **14** (Suppl.), S149–S150.

—— Nomura, Y. (1990) 'The pathophysiology of the Rett syndrome from the standpoint of polysomnography.' *Brain and Development*, **12**, 55–60.

Steffenburg, S (1991) 'Neuropsychiatric assessment of children with autism: a population-based study.' *Developmental Medicine and Child Neurology*, **33**, 495–511.

Suzuki, H., Hirayama, Y., Sakuragawa, N., Arima, M. (1989) 'Progression of CT scan findings in Rett syndrome.' *No To Hattatsu*, **21**, 321–326. *(Japanese.)*

Wagner, H.J. (1986) 'Rett syndrome: positron emission tomography (PET) studies.' *American Journal of Medical Genetics*, **24** (Suppl. 1), 211–224.

Yoshikawa, H., Fueki, N., Suzuki, H., Sakuragawa, N., Masaaki, I. (1991) 'Cerebral blood flow and oxygen metabolism in Rett syndrome.' *Journal of Child Neurology*, **6**, 237–242.

Zilbovicius, M., Raynaud, C., Rancurel, G. (1989) 'Regional cerebral blood flow measured by SPECT in Pick's disease.' *Journal of Cerebral Blood Flow and Metabolism*, **9** (Suppl. 1), 521. *(Abstract.)*

9
NEUROPATHOLOGY AND NEUROCHEMISTRY

Anders Oldfors, Patrick Sourander and Alan K. Percy

Introduction

Major emphasis has been devoted to demonstrating morphological and biochemical abnormalities in biological samples from individuals affected with Rett syndrome. However, in view of the significant motor and cognitive dysfunction demonstrated already in early childhood by girls with RS, the findings on neuropathological and neurochemical examinations are rather modest. So far, these studies have failed to produce a marker which would allow for definitive diagnosis. In this chapter we summarize the available information on neuropathology and neurochemistry in RS and suggest areas for future research.

Neuropathology

Macroscopic changes

The major and consistent macroscopic change of the CNS in RS is a reduction in the size and weight of the brain. The weight reduction may vary between 12 and 41 per cent below levels of age-matched controls (Rett 1977; Harding *et al.* 1985; Missliwetz and Depastas 1985; Jellinger and Seitelberger 1986; Jellinger *et al.* 1988; Oldfors *et al.* 1988, 1990) and appears to increase with duration of the disease (Table 9.1). The reduction of brain volume affects all parts of the brain, with mild reduction of cortical thickness and slight internal hydrocephalus. In one case the cerebellum was reported to be proportionately large compared to the cerebral hemispheres (Harding *et al.* 1985), but this was not found in another study on the cerebellar changes (Oldfors *et al.* 1988, 1990).

Microscopic changes

CEREBRAL CORTEX

The cerebral cortex shows no major changes when examined by conventional light microscopy. A minor reduction in the number of neurons and slight astrogliosis have been observed in some cases. Microdysgenesis, manifested as the presence of nerve cells, some resembling Cajal–Retzius cells, in the subpial molecular layer of the frontal cortex was described in three cases (Jellinger and Seitelberger 1986, Jellinger *et al.* 1988). Other signs of microdysgenesis, *e.g.* clustering of cortical neurons and subcortical heterotopic nerve cells, have not been reported. Electron microscopic studies have revealed an increase in the amount of pigment with the morphological characteristics of lipofuscin in neurons, astrocytes and pericytes (Jellinger and Seitelberger 1986, Jellinger *et al.* 1988, Papadimitriou *et al.* 1988). In the frontal cortex occasional abnormal neurites have been described, consisting of circular profiles filled with lysosomes and laminated bodies (Jellinger *et al.* 1988). In another study, membrane-bound electron-dense inclusions with a distinct lamellar and granular substructure were described in neurons and oligodendroglia (Papadimitriou *et al.* 1988). Preliminary results from studies on cerebral cortex, using a Golgi technique, indicate that decreased dendritic branching may be of importance in RS (Armstrong 1992).

WHITE MATTER

Mild, inconsistent spongy changes of the cerebral and cerebellar white matter, optic nerves, and myelinated fibre tracts of the brainstem tegmentum have been reported (Rett 1977, Jellinger and Seitelberger 1986, Jellinger *et al.* 1988). Papadimitriou *et al.* (1988) reported pale myelin staining and thin myelin sheaths, and a few axons, which showed accumulations of mitochondria and aggregates of autophagosomes. Except for an increase in hypertrophic astrocytes (Papadimitriou *et al.* 1988), there is no astroglial reaction in the cerebral white matter (Jellinger and Seitelberger 1986, Jellinger *et al.* 1988). Cerebellum on the other hand shows astrogliosis of the white matter, which increases with age (Oldfors *et al.* 1990). The white matter of the spinal cord showed marked gliosis in two young women who died at 20 and 30 years of age (Oldfors *et al.* 1988). Myelination of the CNS appears not to be defective or delayed (Jellinger and Seitelberger 1986, Jellinger *et al.* 1988).

BASAL GANGLIA AND THALAMUS

Ultrastructural examination of the caudate nucleus has shown reactive or degenerative axonal swellings packed with large mitochondria, dense granular bodies, membranous, multilamellar or zebra-like bodies, and disintegrating mitochondria. In the striatum and thalamus there was accumulation of lipofuscin in the cytoplasm of neurons and, less often, in astrocytes and oligodendroglia. The number of astrocytes was found to be slightly increased in the striatum (Jellinger and Seitelberger 1986, Jellinger *et al.* 1988). Kitt *et al.* (1990) reported that the basal forebrain neurons are reduced in size in RS.

MESENCEPHALON, PONS AND MEDULLA OBLONGATA

Morphometric studies of the cholinergic nucleus basalis of Meynert and of the serotonergic nucleus dorsalis raphe, evaluating the total number of neurons and the neuronal densities in two cases showed no differences from age-matched controls (Jellinger and Seitelberger 1986).

Several reports have described changes in the substantia nigra. A consistent morphological change, except in very young patients, is hypopigmentation of the zona compacta of substantia nigra due to the presence of many neurons with a

TABLE 9.1

Major morphological changes in the CNS in Rett syndrome

Patient	ES	PC		US 36	TF	WH	MB		GB	S35		HG	SG	PE	US6	S12	S21
Age (yrs)	4	6	6	7	8	11	11	11	12	12	14	15	15	17	17	20	30
Reference*	a	a	b	c	a	a	a	d	a	c	e	a	a	a	c	c,f	c,f
Brain weight (g)		1000	†	1050	1070	840	840	777	910	900	830	1050	950	920	920	1050	980
Normal brain weight (g)**		1210		1250	1260	1270	1270	1270	1280	1280	1285	1285	1285	1290	1290	1300	1300
Cerebral cortex																	
Atrophy	−	+	−		+	++	++	+?	+	+	+	++	+	−			
Gliosis	+	++			+	+	++		−		−	+	−	−		−	+
Microdysgenesis	−	Frontal	−		Frontal	−	−		−		−	−	Frontal	−		−	−
Hypopigmentation of substantia nigra	−	−	−		++	+++	+++	++?	++		++	+++	++	+++		+++	+++
White matter																	
Spongiosis	++	++	−		++	++	++		+			+					
Gliosis	+	−	+		−	−	−	−	−			+	−	−		−	−
Cerebellum																	
Atrophy				+						++					++	+++	++++
Gliosis				+						++	+				++	+++	++++
Spinal cord																	
Gliosis of white and grey matter																+++	+++

*References: a—Jellinger et al. (1988); b—Papadimitriou et al. (1988); c—Oldfors et al. (1990); d—Missliwetz and Depastas (1985); e—Harding et al. (1985); f—Oldfors et al. (1988).

**Lemire et al. (1975).

†Brain biopsy.

Degree: − none; + very mild; ++ mild; +++ moderate; ++++ marked.

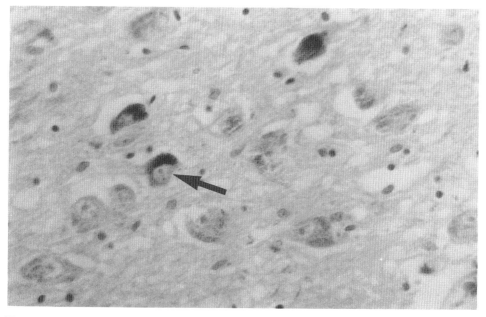

Fig. 9.1. Zona compacta of substantia nigra of 20-year-old woman with RS. Only a few nerve cells show normal pigmentation *(arrow)*, while the majority show reduced number of neuromelanin granula. (Haematoxylin–eosin.)

reduced amount of neuromelanin (Rett 1977, Harding *et al.* 1985, Missliwetz and Depastas 1985, Jellinger and Seitelberger 1986, Jellinger *et al.* 1988, Oldfors *et al.* 1988) (Fig. 9.1). The ultrastructure of the neuromelanin is normal (Jellinger and Seitelberger 1986, Jellinger *et al.* 1988), and there are no or few signs of neuronal degeneration and pigment phagocytosis (Harding *et al.* 1985, Jellinger and Seitelberger 1986, Jellinger *et al.* 1988). Pigmentation of the locus ceruleus appears normal (Jellinger and Seitelberger 1986). Except for minimal spongy changes in white matter the brainstem has not been reported to show any changes.

CEREBELLUM

The cerebellar cortex appears to be more severely affected than the cerebral cortex. In a separate study on the cerebellum in five patients aged 7 to 30 years, the cerebellar cortex displayed general loss of nerve cells in the granular cell layer, the Purkinje cell layer and the molecular cell layer, and there was an accompanying astrogliosis (Oldfors *et al.* 1990). The atrophy was focally accentuated, and was occasionally severe in several adjacent folia (Figs 9.2, 9.3). The atrophy, which was minor in the youngest subject, increased with age, and was generally more pronounced in the tips of the folia. The white matter showed loss of myelinated nerve fibres, and there was a corresponding and in some cases severe astrogliosis, which was most marked around blood vessels. The dentate nucleus showed loss of

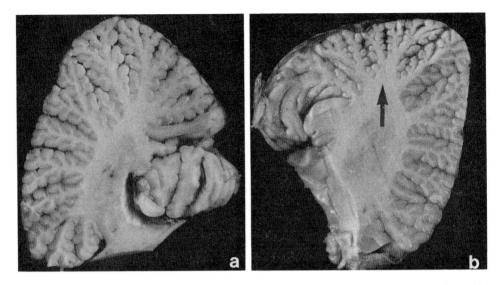

Fig. 9.2. Section through the cerebellar hemispheres of two women with RS, aged 30 years *(a)* and 20 years *(b)*. Note marked general atrophy of folia in *(a)* and focal atrophy of folia in *(b)*. (Reproduced by permission from Oldfors *et al.* 1990)

nerve cells and astrogliosis. The two oldest patients had been treated with phenytoin, which may have contributed to the morphological changes, but atrophy and gliosis increased with age also in the patients without phenytoin treatment. Other authors have reported inconsistent spongy changes in the cerebellar white matter (Rett 1977, Jellinger and Seitelberger 1986).

SPINAL CORD

The spinal cord was examined in two adult subjects, aged 20 and 30 years, with severe scoliosis and cachexia (Oldfors *et al.* 1988). Gliosis of both grey and white matter and loss of spinal ganglion nerve cells, with formation of residual nodules of Nageotte, were reported. Frequent ovoid argyrophilic bodies were present at all levels in the anterior horns (Fig. 9.4). The significance of this finding is difficult to establish, since they have been reported to occur at the lumbosacral level in most adults (Smith 1955). In the two RS patients reported by Oldfors *et al.* (1988) they occurred at all levels of the spinal cord and were not observed in other age-matched patients, which may indicate a degenerative change in the RS patients. The motor neurons appeared to be reduced in number at some levels, but no ongoing degenerative changes of the motor neurons were observed. In the white matter some of the axons of the long ascending and descending tracts demonstrated distorted and enlarged profiles after silver impregnation and after immunohisto-chemical staining of neurofilaments.

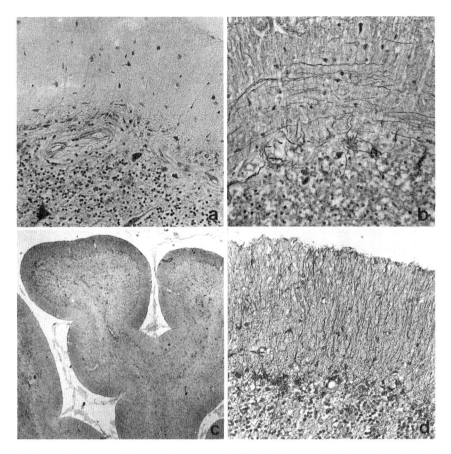

Fig. 9.3. Cerebellar cortex of 30-year-old woman with RS. *(a)* Absence of Purkinje cells and marked loss of granular cells. (Luxol fast blue–cresyl violet.) *(b)* Total loss of Purkinje cells but remnants of baskets. (Palmgren silver impregnation.) *(c, d)* Proliferation of Bergmann glia and radiating glial filaments through the molecular cell layer. (Glial fibrillary acidic protein–immuno staining.) (Reproduced by permission from Oldfors *et al*. 1990.)

PERIPHERAL NERVES

The morphological changes observed in peripheral nerves have usually been of minor degree. In five studied sural nerve biopsies of patients with RS, Haas and Love (1988) found degenerative and occasional regenerative changes in all cases including the youngest patient, who was normally nourished and fully ambulatory. Jellinger *et al*. (1990) studied peripheral nerves in five RS girls. Quantitative analysis of myelinated fibres in two sural nerve biopsy specimens from girls aged 3 and 17 years, respectively, showed redistribution of fibre sizes with preservation of thick myelinated fibres and an increase in small myelinated and unmyelinated fibres. In the 17-year-old and in another girl aged 9 years there were increased

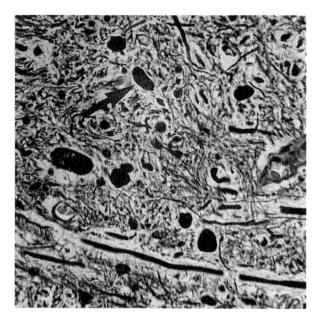

Fig. 9.4. Argyrophilic bodies *(arrow)* in anterior horn of spinal cord in 20-year-old woman with RS. (Palmgren silver impregnation.)

amounts of neurofilaments in some axons, and some axons with thin myelin sheaths suggestive of remyelination of regenerating axons were also observed. Specimens from two girls who died at an advanced stage of disease, one with severe cachexia, at 11 and 17 years respectively, showed minimal reduction of myelinated fibres, but increased numbers of small unmyelinated fibres arranged in clusters. The changes observed by Jellinger *et al.* were suggestive of mild distal axonopathy. Wakai *et al.* (1990) investigated sural nerve biopsies of three patients aged 6 to 7 years. They found many Pi-granules and some swollen mitochondria in Schwann cells in addition to sporadic bands of Büngner and onion bulb formations. Morphometric analysis showed a reduction in the number of large myelinated fibres.

SKELETAL MUSCLE

The results of enzyme histochemical and electron microscopic investigations of skeletal muscle have been reported in several studies. The observed pathological changes have usually been non-specific and highly variable. They include atrophy of type 1 fibres (Haas and Love 1988), type 2 fibres (Dieler *et al.* 1990) or general atrophy (Tulinius *et al.* 1991), as well as disorganization of myofibrils (Jellinger *et al.* 1990) and the presence of tubular structures and concentric laminated bodies in occasional muscle fibres (Jellinger *et al.* 1988, 1990; Eeg-Olofsson *et al.* 1990). Swollen mitochondria, sometimes dumb-bell shaped, have been reported by several authors (Eeg-Olofsson *et al.* 1988, 1990; Ruch *et al.* 1989; Wakai *et al.*

1990). Significant mitochondrial changes were rejected by others (Jellinger *et al.* 1990, Tulinius *et al.* 1991). In one report (Dieler *et al.* 1990), electron-dense deposits in endothelial cells of muscle capillaries were observed in one case. Changes suggestive of denervation appear not to be frequent (Jellinger *et al.* 1990, Wakai *et al.* 1990).

Neurochemistry

Neurochemical investigations in RS have followed a number of lines, the majority of which have occurred within the last decade. The early studies were guided by the prominent movement disorder displayed by girls with RS. Elements of this movement disorder inlude stereotypic movements and disordered breathing patterns during wakefulness, motor apraxia and bradykinesia. Based upon these observations, initial emphasis was placed on examination of the monoamine neurotransmitters. These studies were developed along two avenues: examination of the monoamines and their metabolites in various brain regions, and examination of the metabolites in cerebrospinal fluid (CSF). The results of these studies as well as subsequent neurochemical analyses are presented in the following sections.

Brain neurochemistry

Neurochemical analyses in the CNS of RS patients were initiated in the early 1980s with an examination of monoamines and their metabolites in the brain of one child with RS who died at the age of 11 years (Riederer *et al.* 1985, Brücke *et al.* 1987). Marked reductions in dopamine were noted in multiple brain regions, particularly in the substantia nigra, the putamen, and the caudate nucleus. Interpretation of these results was tempered by the prominent nutritional problems experienced by this child. Subsequent analyses on a series of brain specimens failed to demonstrate the diffuse reduction of dopamine in multiple brain regions but did confirm substantial diminution of dopamine and its metabolite, homovanillic acid, of serotonin and its metabolite, 5-hydroxyindoleacetic acid, and of noradrenaline in the substantia nigra (Lekman *et al.* 1989). These changes appeared to increase with age, suggesting that they may have represented a secondary effect. In a separate study, Wenk *et al.* (1991) also noted a reduction in dopamine in several cortical regions and the putamen. In the same study, these investigators noted reduced levels of choline acetyltransferase activity, particularly in the thalamus, and normal binding of a ligand for high affinity choline uptake sites except in the putamen.

The prominent breathing abnormalities during wakefulness and the reports of sudden death in some children with RS prompted an analysis of ß-endorphins in CSF (see below). Based on the results of this study, tissue levels of ß-endorphins in three brain regions from a single child were compared to those of an age-matched control: ß-endorphin levels were elevated substantially in the thalamus, moderately in the cerebellum and were similar to the control value in the cerebral cortex (Jellinger *et al.* 1988). No evidence of attempts to substantiate these results in additional brain samples is available.

93

Analysis of complex lipids in the cerebrum and cerebellum revealed no major abnormality in the important membrane lipids with the exception of temporal white matter and specific gangliosides (Lekman *et al.* 1991*a,b*). Values for phospholipids in cerebral grey and white matter and in the cerebellum were similar to those obtained from appropriate controls. Similarly, the important myelin lipids galactosylceramide and sulphatide were normal except in temporal white matter. Values for lipid-bound sialic acid, a measure of total ganglioside content, were normal. However, analysis of the individual gangliosides revealed a selective reduction in those associated with axonal terminals and synaptic connections, *viz.* GD1a and GT1b. Whether these findings are related to the primary defect in RS or represent secondary changes is the subject of current investigations. In particular, the reduction of GD1a, a ganglioside prominently arrayed in nerve terminals, could be associated with disordered synaptogenesis.

CSF studies

By virtue of greater accessibility, the number and variety of neurochemical studies of the CSF is substantially greater than those of solid tissues. The initial reports focused on the biogenic amine metabolites. These early investigations demonstrated a reduction in the dopamine metabolite homovanillic acid (HVA) and in the norepinephrine metabolite hydroxymethoxyphenyl glycol (HMPG) in CSF obtained at lumbar puncture (Zoghbi *et al.* 1985). A subsequent study employing a larger sample also noted significant reduction in the serotonin metabolite 5-hydroxyindoleacetic acid (Zoghbi *et al.* 1989). However, reports from other laboratories (including an equally large series from Sweden) failed to corroborate these findings (Perry *et al.* 1988, Lekman *et al.* 1989, Campos-Castelló *et al.* 1991). Indeed, in the largest sample collected to date, data from more than 70 girls with RS, collated by one of the present authors (A.K.P., unpublished), have demonstrated a significant reduction only for the norepinephrine metabolite HMPG and only in the age group from 2 to 4 years. Thus, initial enthusiasm regarding a possible abnormality in the monoamine neurotransmitter system and the possibility of utilizing CSF for diagnosis was blunted.

Biopterin, an essential cofactor in the formation of dopamine and serotonin, was also examined in CSF (Zoghbi *et al.* 1989). Compared to levels in age-matched controls, CSF biopterin levels in girls with RS were significantly elevated. However, subsequent studies failed to demonstrate any abnormalities in the critical element, tetrahydrobiopterin, or in the relevant reductase required for its formation. Thus, the significance of this observation and its relevance to RS is questionable.

As stated above, ß-endorphin levels have been examined in the CSF of girls with RS (Brase *et al.* 1989, Budden *et al.* 1990, Nielsen *et al.* 1991). These studies were prompted by the significant breathing abnormalities experienced by many of the girls during wakefulness as well as by the occurrence of unexplained sudden death in some.

Reduced CSF ß-endorphin levels were reported by Genazzini *et al.* (1989). Interpretation of these data was complicated due to the use of children with leukaemia as controls. However, a recent study by Myer *et al.* (1992) showed that ß-endorphin levels were substantially elevated above those of age-matched controls in over 90 per cent of the 150 samples analyzed. Similar elevations were noted in children with apparently life-threatening episodes (near-miss sudden infant death syndrome) and in other CNS disorders (as reviewed by Myer *et al.* 1992). Thus, the specificity of ß-endorphin elevation is lacking for RS.

Reports of the mitochondrial abnormalities described above led to examination of lactate and pyruvate concentrations in both blood and CSF. Studies in blood (Haas *et al.* 1986, Philippart 1986) failed to demonstrate consistent abnormalities, although in selected instances mild elevations of lactate and/or pyruvate have been reported. Preliminary information on a large series of CSF samples (Matsuishi, personal communication) indicates significant elevation in lactate and pyruvate. However, after segregating the data with respect to the presence of hyperventilation or apnoea, the lactate and pyruvate elevations were seen only in the girls who demonstrated the breathing abnormalities. Once again the findings could be interpreted as secondary.

Direct measurement of respiratory chain enzymes has been carried out in a limited number of muscle biopsies. However, no consistent pattern of reduction was noted (Coker and Melnyk 1991).

As stated above, abnormalities in specific gangliosides in the cerebrum and cerebellum have been described. Extension of these studies to CSF has been conducted in a small series (Svennerholm, personal communication). Preliminary information indicates that similar reductions are not sufficiently consistent at present to allow the use of this technique for diagnostic purposes.

Commentary

What inferences can be made from analysis of the neuropathology and neurochemistry in RS? In the first case, marked morphological abnormalities in neocortical neurons or in white matter have not been reported. The neurochemical findings with regard to complex lipids are consistent with these observations. Namely, the content of myelin lipids is normal, and the overall content of gangliosides, a measure of the neuronal pool, is also normal.

Morphological examination of the nervous system in RS has revealed two major and consistent neuropathological changes. These are hypopigmentation of the zona compacta of the substantia nigra and diffuse and progressive reduction in brain size.

Hypopigmentation of the zona compacta of the substantia nigra is due to a reduction in the number of neuromelanin granules in many of the nerve cells without loss of nerve cells. Pigmentation of the substantia nigra develops during the fifth to 15th year of life. Pigmentation of the zona compacta of the substantia nigra in girls with RS resembles that of normal but considerably younger individuals

(Jellinger and Seitelberger 1986). The significance of the reduced pigmentation is unknown, although reduced levels of the biogenic amines, dopamine, serotonin, and noradrenaline, have been found on biochemical investigation of the substantia nigra of adult but not of young patients with RS (Lekman *et al.* 1989). The dopaminergic neurons of the substantia nigra have their nerve terminals in the striatum. The relation between reactive and degenerative axonal changes described in the caudate nucleus (Jellinger and Seitelberger 1986) and hypopigmentation of the substantia nigra is unknown. However, no reduction in the amount of dopamine was found in the caudate nucleus (Lekman *et al.* 1989).

The severe reduction of brain weight seen in RS patients aged 6 to 7 years when no or only minor astrogliosis is present indicates that hypoplasia rather than atrophy is the cause, since astrogliosis is considered a sensitive marker for CNS atrophy (Herva *et al.* 1988). At older ages (20 to 30 years) the increasing astrogliosis together with loss of nerve cells indicates an additional atrophy. The cause of this hypoplasia and atrophy is unknown. While it is highly speculative, one could postulate that the diffuse reduction in brain size could correlate with the reduction in specific brain gangliosides known to be associated with axons and synaptic connections. This would fall in line with the working hypothesis that RS is a developmental disorder in which the principal neurobiological event is a failure to elaborate critical neuronal networks during the later phases of gestation and the period of early infancy (Hagberg *et al.* 1992). This is a testable hypothesis requiring careful morphometric analysis and study of the quality and quantity of neuronal connections. These areas of investigation would appear to be appropriate targets for future study in RS.

REFERENCES

Armstrong, D.D. (1992) 'The neuropathology of Rett syndrome.' *Brain and Development.* **14** (Suppl.), S89–S98.
Brase, D.A., Myer, E.D., Dewey, W.L. (1989) 'Minireview: Possible hyperendorphinergic patho-physiology of the Rett syndrome.' *Life Sciences*, **45**, 359–366.
Brücke, T., Sofic, E., Killian, W., Rett, A., Riederer, P. (1987) 'Reduced concentrations and increased metabolism of biogenic amines in a single case of Rett syndrome: a postmortem brain study.' *Journal of Neural Transmission*, **68**, 315–324.
Budden, S.S., Myer, E.C., Butler, I.J. (1990) 'Cerebrospinal fluid studies in the Rett syndrome: biogenic amines and ß-endorphins.' *Brain and Development*, **12**, 81–84.
Campos-Castelló, J., De Yébenes, J.G., Mena, M.A., García, F.O. (1991) 'Cerebrospinal fluid concentration of homovanillic acid and 5-hydroxyindoleacetic acid in patients with Rett syndrome.' *International Pediatrics*, **6**, 340–342.
Coker, S.B., Melnyk, A.R. (1991) 'Rett syndrome and mitochondrial enzyme deficiencies.' *Journal of Child Neurology*, **6**, 164–166.
Dieler, R., Schröder, J.M., Reddemann, K. (1990) 'Electron-dense lipidic capillary deposits in Rett syndrome.' *Acta Neuropathologica*, **79**, 573–578.
Eeg-Olofsson, O., Al-Zuhair, A.G.H., Teebi, A.S., Al-Essa, M.M.N. (1988) 'Abnormal mitochondria in the Rett syndrome.' *Brain and Development*, **10**, 260–262.
—— —— —— Daoud, A.S., Zaki, M., Besisso, M.S., Al-Essa, M.M.N. (1990) 'Rett syndrome: a mitochondrial disease?' *Journal of Child Neurology*, **5**, 210–214.

Genazzani, A.R., Zappella, M., Nalin, A., Hayek, Y., Facchinetti, F. (1989) 'Reduced cerebrospinal fluid ß-endorphin levels in Rett syndrome.' *Child's Nervous System*, **5**, 111–113.

Haas, R.H., Love, S. (1988) 'Peripheral nerve findings in Rett syndrome.' *Journal of Child Neurology*, **3** (Suppl.), S25–S30.

—— Rice, M.A., Trauner, D.A., Merrit, T.A. (1986) 'Therapeutic effects of a ketogenic diet in Rett syndrome.' *American Journal of Medical Genetics*, **24** (Suppl. 1), 225–246.

Hagberg, B., Naidu, S., Percy, A.K. (1992) 'Tokyo symposium on Rett syndrome: neurobiological approach.' *Brain and Development*, **14** (Suppl.), S151–S153.

Harding, B.N., Tudway, A.J.C., Wilson, J. (1985) 'Neuropathological studies in a child showing some features of the Rett syndrome.' *Brain and Development*, **7**, 342–344.

Herva, R., Conradi, N.G., Kalimo, H., Leisti, J., Sourander, P. (1988) 'A syndrome of multiple congenital contractures: neuropathological analysis on five fatal cases.' *American Journal of Medical Genetics*, **29**, 67–76.

Jellinger, K., Seitelberger, F. (1986) 'Neuropathology of Rett syndrome.' *American Journal of Medical Genetics*, **1** (Suppl.), 259–288.

—— Armstrong, D., Zoghbi, H.Y., Percy, A.K. (1988) 'Neuropathology of Rett syndrome.' *Acta Neuropathologica*, **76**, 142–158.

—— Grisold, W., Armstrong, D., Rett, A. (1990) 'Peripheral nerve involvement in the Rett syndrome.' *Brain and Development*, **12**, 109–114.

Kitt, C.A., Troncoso, J.C., Price, D.L., Naidu, S., Moser, H.W. (1990) 'Pathological changes in substantia nigra and basal forebrain neurons in Rett syndrome.' *Annals of Neurology*, **28**, 416–417.

Lekman, A., Witt-Engerström, I., Gottfries, J., Hagberg, B.A., Percy, A.K., Svennerholm, L. (1989) 'Rett syndrome: biogenic amines and metabolites in postmortem brain.' *Pediatric Neurology*, **5**, 357–362.

—— Hagberg, B.A., Svennerholm, L.T. (1991*a*) 'Membrane cerebral lipids in Rett syndrome.' *Pediatric Neurology*, **7**, 186–190.

—— —— —— (1991*b*) 'Altered cerebellar ganglioside pattern in Rett syndrome.' *Neurochemistry International*, **19**, 505–509.

Lemire, R.J., Loeser, J.D., Leech, R.W., Alvord, E.C. (1975) *Normal and Abnormal Development of the Human Nervous System.* New York and London: Harper & Row.

Missliwetz, J., Depastas, G. (1985) 'Forensic problems in Rett syndrome.' *Brain and Development*, **7**, 326–328.

Myer, E.C., Tripathi, H.L., Brase, D.A., Dewey, W.L. (1992) 'Elevated CSF betaendorphin immunoreactivity in Rett's syndrome; report of 158 cases and comparison with leukemic children.' *Neurology*, **42**, 357–360.

Nielsen, J.B., Bach, F.W., Buchholt, J., Lou, H. (1991) 'Cerebrospinal fluid ß-endorphin in Rett syndrome.' *Developmental Medicine and Child Neurology*, **33**, 406–411.

Oldfors, A., Hagberg, B., Nordgren, H., Sourander, P., Witt-Engerström, I. (1988) 'Rett syndrome: spinal cord neuropathology.' *Pediatric Neurology*, **4**, 172–174.

—— Sourander, P., Armstrong, D.L., Percy, A.K., Witt-Engerström, I., Hagberg, B.A. (1990) 'Rett syndrome: cerebellar pathology.' *Pediatric Neurology*, **6**, 310–314.

Papadimitriou, J.M., Hockey, A., Tan, N., Masters, C.L. (1988) 'Rett syndrome: abnormal membrane-bound lamellated inclusions in neurons and oligodendroglia.' *American Journal of Medical Genetics*, **29**, 365–368.

Perry, T.L., Dunn, H.G., Ho, H.H., Crichton, J.U. (1988) 'Cerebrospinal fluid values for monoamine metabolites, γ-aminobutyric acid, and other amino compounds in Rett syndrome.' *Journal of Pediatrics*, **112**, 234–238.

Philippart, M. (1986) 'Clinical recognition of Rett syndrome.' *American Journal of Medical Genetics*, **24** (Suppl. 1), 111–118.

Rett, A. (1977) 'Cerebral atrophy associated with hyperammonaemia.' *In*: Vinken, P.J., Bruyn, G.W. (Eds) *Handbook of Clinical Neurology. Vol. 29: Metabolic and Deficiency Diseases of the Nervous System, Part 3.* Amsterdam: North Holland.

Riederer, P., Brücke, T., Sofic, E., Kienzl, E., Schnecker, K., Schay, V., Kruzik, P., Killian, W., Rett, A. (1985) 'Neurochemical aspects of the Rett syndrome.' *Brain and Development*, **7**, 351–360.

Ruch, A., Kurczynski, T.W., Velasco, M.E. (1989) 'Mitochondrial alterations in Rett syndrome.' *Pediatric Neurology*, **5**, 320–323.

97

Smith, M.C. (1955) 'Argyrophilic bodies in the human spinal cord.' *Journal of Neurology, Neurosurgery and Psychiatry*, **18**, 13–16.

Tulinius, M., Holme, E., Kristiansson, B., Larsson, N-G., Oldfors, A. (1991) 'Mitochondrial encephalomyopathies in children. I. Biochemical and morphological investigations.' *Journal of Pediatrics*, **119**, 242–250.

Wakai, S., Kameda, K., Ishikawa, Y., Miyamoto, S., Nagaoka, M., Okabe, M., Minami, R., Tachi, N. (1990) 'Rett syndrome: findings suggesting axonopathy and mitochondrial abnormalities.' *Pediatric Neurology*, **6**, 339–343.

Wenk, G.L., Naidu, S., Cassanova, M.F., Kitt, C.A., Moser, H. (1991) 'Altered neurochemical markers in Rett syndrome.' *Neurology*, **41**, 1753–1736.

Zoghbi, H.Y., Percy, A.K., Glaze, D.G., Butler, I.J., Riccardi, V.M. (1985) 'Reduction of biogenic amine levels in the Rett syndrome.' *New England Journal of Medicine*, **313**, 921–924.

—— Milstien, S., Butler, I.M., Smith, E.O'B., Kaufman, S., Glaze, D.G., Percy, A.K. (1989) 'Cerebrospinal fluid biogenic amines and biopterin in Rett syndrome.' *Annals of Neurology*, **25**, 56–60.

10
GENETIC CONSIDERATIONS AND CLUES FROM MOLECULAR GENETICS

Maria Anvret, Jan Wahlström and Hans-Olof Åkesson

Introduction

Although there is as yet no conclusive proof, the evidence for Rett syndrome being a genetic disorder is today convincing. It is supported by the existence of a few familial cases, and by concordance among monozygotic (MZ) female twins and discordance among dizygotic (DZ) twins (Zoghbi 1988). Because only girls are affected, an X-linked dominant inheritance due to a new mutation in each case, non-viable in males, has been suggested (Hagberg *et al.* 1983). This hypothesis is partly supported by the discovery of two translocations involving the X chromosome (Journel *et al.* 1990, Zoghbi *et al.* 1990a), but not by the presence of familial cases. However, molecular genetic studies on the X chromosome have so far been disappointing. Genealogical studies have also indicated that pattern of inheritance other than X-linked dominance may be of importance in RS (Åkesson *et al.* 1992).

Current knowledge concerning the inheritance of RS is reviewed in this chapter.

Twin data

Twin studies are one way to determine whether or not a disease is genetically transmitted, but they tell nothing about the mode of inheritance. In a fully penetrant dominant genetic trait one would expect all MZ twins to be concordant as they have all their genes in common. Half or less of the DZ twins would be concordant, having common genes in the same proportion as non-twin sibs. However, this is seldom the case. A higher frequency of concordant MZ than DZ twins would indicate the possibility of an hereditary trait, since if a disorder is caused only by environmental factors MZ and DZ twins raised in the same environment would be concordant to the same degree.

The International Rett Syndrome Association (IRSA) register includes seven concordant MZ and 11 discordant DZ twin pairs (Hunter, personal communication). Of the DZ twin pairs, four are female/female and seven are female/male. The finding of only concordant MZ twins is strong evidence for RS being an hereditary disorder. However, the twins in the register are clinically heterogeneous and any conclusion must therefore be drawn carefully.

A dominant mutation in one DZ twin does not affect the co-twin. The only ways a mutation could affect both individuals in a DZ twin pair would be if the mother has a germ cell line mutation or if there is a mutation in each twin. The finding that the DZ twins known so far are discordant supports the dominant X-linked mutation hypothesis. One would also expect a lower number of DZ twin pairs with one RS-affected girl, since the intrauterine death of any male DZ twin would either trigger a spontaneous abortion of both fetuses or lead to the later birth of a singleton girl, in which case the twin gestation might not be identified. Were a lower than expected frequency of discordant DZ twin pairs with RS to be found in an epidemiological study of twins, this would also support a dominant X-linked inheritance. However, the population needed for such a study is very large, making it unfeasible.

Family studies
The segregation pattern of a trait in families makes it possible to determine whether it is genetic. A recessively inherited disease is found in 25 per cent of the children but not in the parents. A dominantly inherited disease is in most cases found in one of the parents and in 50 per cent of the children. The recent report of a family in which RS has been transmitted from mother to daughter strongly supports a dominant inheritance (Witt Engerström and Forslund 1992). Furthermore there are now eight known sibships which include two sisters with RS. Two of these affected pairs are half-sisters. RS has also been diagnosed in two generations of two families in an aunt and niece (Anvret *et al.* 1990; Hagberg *et al.* 1990; Clarke, personal communication). However, considering that more than 2000 females with RS have now been identified, there are far too few first grade relatives with the syndrome to fulfil the criteria for either simple recessive or dominant transmission.

Genetic counselling
The few familial cases observed are of importance in the genetic counselling of families with a child with RS. The risk of having a second girl with RS is increased but is still very low, probably less than 0.4 per cent. This figure is based on the assumption of eight family cases among at least 2000 RS patients in the IRSA register. Family cases are most likely almost always reported to the register, whereas isolated cases may not be, so the true risk is probably lower. As no marker has yet been found for the disease, prenatal diagnosis is not possible.

Cytogenetic findings
Structural chromosome aberrations such as translocations may segregate in families, both in sibships and between different generations. We have observed two such aberrations in girls with RS: a small duplication on chromosome 6 [dup(6)(p11.2)] (Wahlström and Anvret 1986), and a balanced translocation between chromosomes 16 and 17 [t(16;17)(p13;q21)]. However, identical aberrations were found in one of the parents in both instances. Such an observation has earlier been taken as evidence that there is no connection between the aberration

and the clinical findings, although recently genetic imprinting has been suggested as a mechanism by which a balanced structural aberration can have clinical significance in the child but not in the parent. In the parent the normal chromosome may be functioning, whereas in the child the translocation chromosome is active due to genetic imprinting. If a gene of importance for the development of RS is located at the breakpoint then the girl will have RS.

A *de novo* balanced translocation is one without loss or gain of cytogenetically identified material and not present in either parent. Although the chromosome aberration is not a direct cause of the disorder, there are other reasons for an interest in it. Assuming a genetic factor behind RS, there must be some kind of defect in the DNA. In some girls, maybe only a single case, this DNA damage could be identified as a structural chromosome aberration and indicate where to look for a possible RS gene.

Structural aberrations involving the X chromosome are of special interest as only girls are affected. Two such translocations have been reported with different breakpoints in the short arm of the X chromosome. Zoghbi *et al.* (1990*a*) described a case of RS with a translocation [46,XX,t(X;3)(p22.11;q13.31)]. The breakpoint on the X chromosome has recently been revised to Xp21.3 by YAC (yeast artificial chromosome) cloning and by the use of radiation hybrid cell lines containing small pieces of Xp (Ellison *et al.* 1992). The other case—46,XX,t(X;22) (p11.22;p11) (Journel *et al.* 1990)—is less convincing, as the mother of the Rett girl has the same translocation but without the Rett phenotype. This may however be explained by different X inactivation patterns or by genetic imprinting in the mother or the father. If so, Journel *et al.* postulate that the gene for RS may be located distally to the breakpoint. These cases are currently being subjected to thorough investigation using molecular genetic methods.

Our observation of a small deletion on the short arm of the X chromosome [del(X)(p22)] in 10 per cent of analysed cells in two separate fibroblast cultures from a girl with RS (Wahlström and Anvret 1986) indicates that the X chromosome is of importance for the understanding of the development of RS.

If RS were a contiguous gene syndrome with a common small deletion, only single cases in each family would be observed. However, no such deletion has been identified and therefore this mechanism for RS seems unlikely.

It is of interest to note that RS has not been found in any individual with a numerical sex chromosome aberration. Any observation of RS in a boy with Klinefelter syndrome (47,XXY) would strongly suggest that the gene for RS is on the X chromosome. RS in a girl with Turner syndrome (45,XO) or triple X syndrome (47,XXX) would also suggest the gene to be on the X chromosome. All male cases showing RS-like phenotypes are also of interest in order to help understand the aetiology of the syndrome.

RS is not caused by any chromosome aberration. It is of great importance, however, to perform cytogenetic investigations using the best possible techniques in all affected girls to detect structural chromosomal changes. RS girls with other malformations or diseases are of special interest for study as a small deletion in a chromosome found in such an individual may include more than the gene for RS and thus cause the other malformations or diseases. The breakpoints involved in any translocation are also of interest as the site for a gene of importance for the development of RS.

Fragile sites

As only girls are affected by RS, great interest has been focused on detecting any aberration on the X chromosome. Using a special culture technique, in which caffeine (2.2mmol/L) was added to the culture medium, we were able to demonstrate that girls with RS had a significantly higher frequency of fragile Xp22 than an age-matched control group (Wahlström *et al.* 1990). Unfortunately, this is a very common fragile site found in most normal people and thus is of no use as a marker for RS. However, the increased frequency found in RS may indicate that further study of this region (using, for example, molecular genetic technology) might be of value. Investigation using other culture media, such as one low in folic acid, revealed no differences between RS girls and controls. A culture depleted of folic acid is of interest in this connection as it is used to detect fragile Xq27.3, the site associated with fragile X syndrome.

Telvi *et al.* (1991) have confirmed the increased frequency of fragile Xp22 in girls with RS. They also found an increased rate of other fragile sites, and concluded that RS is a chromosomal breakage syndrome.

Genealogical studies

In a Swedish study (Åkesson *et al.* 1992) we have observed a highly significant increased rate of consanguinity among both paternal and maternal ancestors of girls with RS. Analyses of parental ages at birth and of birth order gave normal results, as expected when a disease is genetically determined. A special finding of interest from this fairly comprehensive study was the fact that the number of male sibs did not significantly differ from the number of female sibs, an observation that does not favour an X-linked dominant transmission with early miscarriage of male fetuses.

In the same study, covering 77 Swedish girls with classical RS, common ancestry was seen in two pairs of affected girls born in completely different parts of Sweden. Furthermore, 39 of the 77 subjects were traced to nine small and separate areas, and for 17 pairs ancestry was even traced to the same farm or homestead. Common origin was observed among both maternal and paternal descendants. This apparent existence of specific 'Rett areas' is supported by our preliminary findings (unpublished) in a genealogical investigation of an additional 18 consecutively found girls with RS diagnosed after the above-mentioned study took place.

Such observations strongly suggest that the primary genetic event that causes RS occurs in earlier generations. They also favour a genetic transmission that is not only mediated by the X chromosome. A second critical factor may be an accumulation of genetic events taking place in successive generations. Such amplifications are known to occur in fragile X syndrome, where an initial amplification of a CGG island within the gene in question must pass through a female to be methylated in order to become expressed (Ying-Hui *et al.* 1991). In the case of RS such an amplification could proceed very slowly, and many generations may pass before it reaches a critical value. The increased frequency of fragile Xp22 may be an instance where such an accumulation of genetic events has taken place in girls with RS.

Molecular genetic studies

The relatively low familial occurrence of RS is a severe limitation when it comes to molecular genetic investigations. These kind of studies are generally based on families where the disorder under study is present in several informative generations or is segregating in many families. By putting the few families together and using several approaches to extract all the available information it is possible to test a few hypotheses. Five avenues of investigation are described:
(1) segregation analysis of the X chromosome in familial cases;
(2) germline mosaicism in the mothers of RS girls;
(3) inactivation–activation pattern of the X chromosome;
(4) characterization of candidate genes of the X chromosome;
(5) mitochondrial DNA analysis.

Segregation analysis of the X chromosome in familial cases
Interest in this area has focused on the short arm of the X chromosome (Xp) because of four different observations: (i) no males with convincing RS have yet been reported; (ii) an increased frequency of the common fragile site Xp22 in girls with RS (see above); (iii) two translocations described involving the short arm of the X chromosome but with different breakpoints (see above); and (iv) an X-linked metabolic defect observed in the enzyme ornithine transcarbamylase (OTC) in some RS families (Thomas *et al.* 1987, 1990; Clark *et al.* 1990).

Segregation analysis of the X chromosome has been performed, in the few family cases available, with polymorphic DNA markers from the X chromosome (Anvret *et al.* 1990). Different approaches were used in order to obtain a complete picture of how different parts of the X chromosomes segregated. Recombinations during the meiotic cell divisions are one important obstacle in such studies. The idea is to analyse regions of the chromosome which are present or not present in the familial RS cases. Discordance for certain regions indicates that a gene or genes of interest are not located in these parts. Concordance for certain regions would support the opposite situation, indicating sites of interest in the search for candidate genes. However, it is not possible to perform regular linkage analysis due to the small number of families with more than one RS girl known. Concordance is only an indication that the region could include genes of interest. The method can in most cases only be used to exclude regions on the chromosomes which are discordant.

To summarize the results of the segregation analyses, almost the whole X chromosome can be excluded except the region at the most distal end of both the long Xq and the short Xp arms of the chromosome. No other chromosome pair has been subjected to this kind of exclusion analysis.

The amount of work needed for this kind of analysis was formerly very great, due to the lack of suitable polymorphic markers. However, the identification of highly variable DNA markers such as VNTR (variable number of tandem repeats) probes (Nakamura *et al.* 1987) and CA repeats (Weber and May 1989, Weber 1990) has made this kind of study possible with more reasonable effort.

Germline mosaicism in the mothers of RS girls
The use of somatic cell hybrids to map the two maternal X chromosomes is similar to regular segregation analysis. The idea behind this is to separate the X chromosomes in order to find out if the mother is mosaic in her germline, which might explain why one daughter develops RS while another does not. It can also to a certain extent explain why the mother carrying a mutation is unaffected and the daughter is not. The mother may carry the mutation in her egg cells but not in her somatic cells, and thus be a carrier for RS without showing clinical signs. The same situation can occur on the paternal side. The most suitable families to test this on are those with two half-sisters with different fathers. Using this approach Archidiacono *et al.* (1991) were able to exclude possible regions of the X chromosome for RS mutations and to show that the two half-sisters in the family studied did not inherit the same alleles for most locations explored. Two regions they could not exclude were those around the OTC locus in Xp21.1 and the translocation breakpoint Xp22.11 (Zoghbi *et al.* 1990*a*), revised to Xp21.3 (Ellison *et al.* 1991) and Xp11.22 (Journel *et al.* 1990), respectively.

Inactivation–activation pattern of the X chromosome
The hypothesis of an extreme lyonization (random X-inactivation) and parental imprinting of a specific X chromosomal region could explain the phenotypic expression of RS among females. This implies a maternal uniparental heterodisomy and paternal nullisomy with a maternal chromosomal duplication. This has been looked for in one case by Benedetti *et al.* (1992); they found no supportive indications, contradicting earlier observations by Zoghbi *et al.* (1990*b*) concerning non-random X-inactivation. Benedetti *et al.* postulated that RS may result from a recent dominant paternal X chromosome mutation: when this is passed to a female child she develops RS, but when passed to a male it is lethal.

This supports our observations in a family with RS in two generations (Anvret *et al.* 1990). We found that the grandpaternal X chromosome was concordant in the niece and aunt with RS. We investigated the inactivation pattern using the X chromosomal marker M27-beta (DXS255) in this family (Anvret and Wahlström 1992*a*). It was found to be random, contradicting earlier findings by Riccardi (1986) and Zoghbi *et al.* (1990*b*). It was further investigated using autopsy material (brain and liver) from two girls. A random pattern of X-inactivation was again noted (personal data, unpublished).

The statement that no male cases are found is questionable. There are reports of males with RS phenotypes (see Chapter 5) but so far these have not been generally accepted as representing true RS.

Characterization of candidate genes on the X chromosome
Genes of the short arm of the X chromosome, for example those coding for OTC, synapsin I and synaptophysin, may explain the genetic background. They are all located within the region not entirely excluded as the locus for RS according to segregation and germline mosaicism studies. OTC has been reported to be defective in some girls with RS (Thomas *et al.* 1987, 1990; Clarke *et al.* 1990), although involvement of the OTC locus could not be supported either by investigation of other RS cases or by molecular genetic analysis (Anvret *et al.* 1990, Archidiacono *et al.* 1991, Ellison *et al.* 1992).

Again, no structural abnormalities have so far been found at the gene loci associated with either synapsin (Xp11.3–Xp11.23) (Yang-Feng *et al.* 1986, Kirchgessner *et al.* 1991) or synaptophysin (Xp11.22–Xp11.23) (Özcelik *et al.* 1990). This does not, however, exclude the possible presence of point mutations within the genes. In order to further investigate this, the chromosomal regions have to be sequenced from patients with RS. These X-linked candidate genes have so far not been found to be responsible for the development of RS.

Mitochondrial DNA analysis
A mitochondrial inheritance was partly supported by the finding in one study of abnormal mitochondrial structures in muscle tissue from RS girls (Eeg-Olofsson *et al.* 1988). However, no other published report has so far lent support to this observation. We have investigated the mitochondrial DNA in autopsy material from two girls. The biopsies were from the liver and brain. No deletions were detected (Anvret *et al.* 1990) in either case. This does not, however, exclude the possibility of point mutations in the mitochondrial DNA.

Discussion
On current knowledge it is still unclear whether RS is an inherited disorder and if so which specific chromosomal region is involved. There are findings both supporting and opposing the involvement of the X chromosome. The hypothesis mostly favoured is an X-linked dominant inheritance which is lethal in males. Neither clinical nor epidemiological data contradict this, but equally no positive molecular evidence has so far been found despite intensive investigation. The finding of families with more than one Rett girl may be explained if RS is caused by a germ cell line mutation in the unaffected mother. The occurrence of RS in two different generations, as in an aunt and niece, must then be explained by two different mutations in the two cases.

There may well be an even more complicated mode of inheritance, with not only involvement of the X chromosome but also an autosomal locus. The X locus may predispose the sex distribution, and the autosomal locus, when mutated, may account for the special syndrome (Johnson 1980). This theory has been partially discussed on a theoretical level by Bühler *et al.* (1990). This kind of transmission has been observed in the inheritance of neurodegeneration in the nematode *Caenorhabditis elegans* (Chalfie and Wolinsky 1990). In this case two genes are involved: when one is mutated neurodegeneration does not occur but when it is demutated it does. This means that one mutation can be inherited without resulting in a syndrome but if the other is also present then the syndrome develops.

Our genealogical and molecular genetic observations support this two mutation model (Anvret and Wahlström 1992*b*). One of the mutations might very well be autosomal. The X chromosome has been extensively analysed (Ellison *et al.* 1992), but because there are so few family cases, regions can only be excluded so far. It is noteworthy that molecular genetic studies have not yet excluded the critical region on the X chromosome where we have found an increased frequency of fragile Xp22. No specific X chromosomal region has been implicated in all cases investigated.

The inheritance of RS is an enigma, and we believe that there is reason to investigate other than simple mendelian inheritance. Developments during the last few years have taught us many new genetic principles, such as fragile sites and genetic imprinting, which have explained some of the inconsistencies observed in the inheritance of other mendelian traits. A new genetic principle could be the answer to the enigma.

REFERENCES

Åkesson, H.O., Hagberg, B., Wahlström, J., Witt Engerström, I. (1992) 'Rett syndrome: a search for gene sources.' *American Journal of Medical Genetics*, **42**, 104–108.
Anvret, M., Wahlström, J., Skogsberg, P., Hagberg, B. (1990) 'Segregation analysis of the X-chromosome in a family with Rett syndrome in two generations.' *American Journal of Medical Genetics*, **37**, 31–35.
——— (1992*a*) 'Reply to Dr Benedetti *et al.*' *American Journal of Medical Genetics*, **44**, 123. (*Letter.*)
——— (1992*b*) 'Genetics of Rett syndrome.' *Brain and Development*, **14** (Suppl.), S101–S103.
Archidiacono, N., Lerone, M., Rocchi, M., Anvret, M., Özcelik, T., Francke, U., Romeo, G. (1991) 'Rett syndrome: exclusion mapping following the hypothesis of germinal mosaicism for new X-linked mutations in the mother of two affected half sisters.' *Human Genetics*, **86**, 604–606.
Benedetti, L., Munnich, A., Melki, J. Tardieu, M., Turleau, C. (1992) 'Parental origin of the X chromosomes in Rett syndrome.' *American Journal of Medical Genetics*, **44**, 121–122. (*Letter.*)
Bühler, E.M., Malik, N.J., Alkan, M. (1990) 'Another model for the inheritance of Rett syndrome.' *American Journal of Medical Genetics*, **36**, 126–131.
Chalfie, M., Wolinsky, E. (1990) 'The identification and suppression of inherited neurodegeneration in *Caenorhabditis elegans*.' *Nature*, **345**, 410–416.
Clarke, A., Gardner-Medwin, D., Richardson, J., McGann, A., Bonham, J.R., Carpenter, K.H., Bhattacharya, S., Haggerty, D., Fleetwood, J.A., Aynsley-Green, A. (1990) 'Abnormalities of carbohydrate metabolism and of OCT gene function in the Rett syndrome.' *Brain and Development*, **12**, 119–124.
Eeg-Olofsson, O., Al-Zuhair, A.G.H., Teebi, A.S., Al-Essa, M.N. (1988) 'Abnormal mitochondria in Rett syndrome.' *Brain and Development*, **10**, 260–262.

Ellison, K.A., Fill, C.P., Terwilliger, J., DeGennaro, L.J., Martin-Gallardo, A., Anvret, M., Percy, A.K., Ott, J., Zoghbi, H. (1992) 'Examination of the X chromosome markers in Rett syndrome: exclusion mapping with a novel variation on multilocus linkage analysis.' *American Journal of Human Genetics*, **50**, 278–287.

Hagberg, B., Aicardi, J., Dias, K., Ramos, O. (1983) 'A progressive syndrome of autism, dementia, ataxia, and loss of purposeful hand use in girls: Rett syndrome: report of 35 cases.' *Annals of Neurology*, **14**, 471–479.

—— Anvret, M., Wahlström, J. (1990) 'Classical Rett syndrome girl with "forme fruste" variant maternal aunt.' *Brain and Development*, **12**, 47–48.

Johnson, W.F. (1980) 'Metabolic interference and the +/–heterozygote. A hypothetical form of simple inheritance which is neither dominant nor recessive.' *American Journal of Human Genetics*, **32**, 374–386.

Journel, H., Melki, J., Turleau, C., Munnich, A., de Grouchy, J. (1990) 'Rett phenotype with X/autosome translocation: possible mapping to the short arm of chromosome X.' *American Journal of Medical Genetics*, **35**, 142–147.

Kirchgessner, C.U., Trofatter, J.A., Mahtani, M.M., Willard, H.F., DeGennaro, L.J. (1991) 'A highly polymorphic dinucleotide repeat on the proximal short arm of the human X chromosome: linkage mapping of the Synapsin 1/A-raf-1 genes.' *American Journal of Human Genetics*, **49**, 184–191.

Nakamura, Y., Leppert, M., O'Connell, P., Wolff, R., Holm, T., Culver, M., Martin, C., Fujimoto, E., Hoff, M., Kumlin, E., *et al.* (1987) 'Variable number of tandem repeat (VNTR) markers for human gene mapping.' *Science*, **235**, 1616–1622.

Özcelik, T., Lafreniere, R.G., Archer, B.T., Johnston, P.A., Willard, H.F., Francke, U., Sudhof, T.C. (1990) 'Synaptophysin: structure of the human gene and assignment to the X chromosome in man and mouse.' *American Journal of Human Genetics*, **47**, 551–561.

Riccardi, V.M. (1986) 'The Rett syndrome: genetics and the future.' *American Journal of Medical Genetics*, **24** (Suppl. 1), 389–402.

Telvi, L., Leboyer, M., Chiron, C., Feingold, J., Pompidou, A., Ponsot, G. (1991) 'The fragile site Xp22 in Rett syndrome as a consequence of a "chromosome breakage syndrome".' *Psychiatric Genetics*, **2**, 57. (*Abstract*.)

Thomas, S., Hjelm, M., Oberholzer, V., Brett, E.M., Wilson, J. (1987) 'Rett's syndrome and ornithine carbamoyltransferase deficiency.' *Lancet*, **2**, 1330–1331.

—— Oberholzer, V., Wilson, J., Hjelm, M. (1990) 'The urea cycle in the Rett syndrome.' *Brain and Development*, **12**, 93–96.

Wahlström, J., Anvret, M. (1986) 'Chromosome findings in the Rett syndrome and a test of a two-step mutation theory.' *American Journal of Medical Genetics*, **24** (Suppl. 1), 361–368.

—— Witt-Engerström, I., Mellquist, L., Anvret, M., Oden, A. (1990) 'The Rett syndrome related to fragile X(p22) in caffeine-induced lymphocyte culture.' *Brain and Development*, **12**, 128–130.

Weber, J.L. (1990) 'Informativeness of human (dC-dA)n(dG-dT)n polymorphisms.' *Genomics*, **7**, 524–530.

—— May, P.E. (1989) 'Abundant class of human DNA polymorphisms which can be typed using the polymerase chain reaction.' *American Journal of Human Genetics*, **44**, 388–396.

Witt Engerström, I., Forslund, M. (1992) 'Mother and daughter with Rett syndrome.' *Developmental Medicine and Child Neurology*, **34**, 1022–1023. (*Letter.*)

Yang-Feng, T.L., DeGennaro, L.J., Francke, U. (1986) 'Genes for synapsin 1, a neuronal phosphoprotein, map to conserved regions of human and murine X chromosomes.' *Proceedings of the National Academy of Science of the USA*, **83**, 8679–8683.

Ying-Hui, F., Kuhl, D.P.A., Pizzuti, A., Pieretti, M., Sutcliffe, J.S., Richards, S., Verkerk, A.J.M.H., Holden, J.J.A., Fenwick, R.G., Warren, S.T., *et al.* (1991) 'Variation of the CGG repeat at the fragile X site results in genetic instability: resolution of the Sherman paradox.' *Cell*, **67**, 1047–1058.

Zoghbi, H.Y. (1988) 'Genetic aspects of Rett syndrome.' *Journal of Child Neurology*, **3** (Suppl.), S76–S78.

—— Ledbetter, D.H., Schultz, R.J., Percy, A.K., Glaze, D.G. (1990a) 'A de novo X;3 translocation in Rett syndrome.' *American Journal of Medical Genetics*, **35**, 148–151.

—— Percy, A.K., Schultz, R.J., Fill, C. (1990b) 'Patterns of X chromosome inactivation in the Rett syndrome.' *Brain and Development*, **12**, 131–135.

11
THERAPY IN RETT SYNDROME: DRUG TRIALS AND FAILURES

Alan K. Percy and Bengt Hagberg

Current therapeutic approaches to girls with RS are directed along the lines of providing habilitation with regard to physical and occupational therapy and communication skills and of providing suitable medication for the management of seizures. Seizure control may be vexing in some instances, but in general is accomplished without major difficulty. Specific medication should be based on clinical seizure type and EEG pattern. However, it is our experience and that of others that carbamazepine is a very effective agent. In addition, sodium valproate has proved to be a suitable alternative. In terms of general health, some children may require special nutritional programmes for maintenance of adequate weight, including in some cases, feeding by gastrostomy tube. Vitamin and cofactor replacement in therapeutic amounts has not been critically evaluated. In particular, pyridoxine merits attention given its pivotal role in neurotransmitter synthesis.

Therapy directed at the fundamental mechanisms underlying RS has failed to produce any substantive improvements, despite the use of multiple different preparations (Rett 1992). In particular, drugs aimed at the monoamine system (Table 11.1), including L-dopa and the dopamine agonists bromocriptine and pergolide, have failed to provide improvement on a consistent basis. Few published reports regarding controlled trials of any of these drugs are available. Instead, most experience is based on open-label trials, and efficacy has been judged by parental reports or clinical observations. Unfortunately, little in the way of objective assessment can be expected from such uncontrolled studies. Our own experience with L-dopa has revealed no consistently favourable effect, with the possible exception of improvement in rigidity which may accompany the stage of late motor deterioration (Stage IV). However, even these observations are not based on controlled conditions.

The most extensive description of clinical trials involves the dopamine agonist bromocriptine. In three reports, Zappella and co-workers described their experience with a total of 12 girls with typical RS and one with forme fruste (Zappella and Genazzani 1986, Zappella 1990, Zappella *et al.* 1990). The latter two studies were conducted under a standardized format during which bromocriptine was provided for six months followed by a two month washout period with the subsequent resumption of the bromocriptine. Improvements in communication and agitation were described, particularly during the first treatment phase; however,

TABLE 11.1

Pharmacological approaches to Rett syndrome

Replacement
        L-dopa/carbidopa
        Tryptophan/tyrosine

Dopamine agonists
        Bromocriptine
        Pergolide

Other aminergic agents
        Selegiline
        Tetrabenazine

Antiepileptic agents
        Carbamazepine
        Sodium valproate

after the washout phase, during which previous behaviours tended to recur, resumption of bromocriptine was not associated with a similar level of improvement. Overall, no dramatic reversal of the motor and behavioural abnormalities typically seen in RS was observed. Nevertheless, these reports can form the basis for future double-blind controlled studies evaluating either bromocriptine or its related agent, pergolide.

In a separate clinical trial, based on the suggestion of deficient neurotransmitter levels in RS, Nielsen *et al.* (1990) attempted neurotransmitter precursor therapy with the amino acids tyrosine (dopamine and noradrenaline) and tryptophan (serotonin) in nine girls. In the first phase, they demonstrated an increase in homovanillic acid (dopamine) and 5-hydroxyindoleacetic acid (serotonin) levels in CSF. Next, utilizing a double-blind crossover strategy, 11 girls were treated in a similar fashion with tyrosine and tryptophan. After eight to ten weeks each of placebo or amino acid therapy, no differences in clinical performances or EEG patterns were noted. In this regard, one of us (B.H.) had earlier noted that tryptophan, administered orally, resulted in improved night-time sleep and less screaming both in girls with RS and in children with infantile neuronal ceroid lipofuscinosis, probably as non-specific effects (unpublished observations).

Reports of elevated levels of β-endorphins in CSF (see Chapter 9) led to the design of a double-blind crossover trial of the opiate antagonist, naltrexone. In the initial report from this study, Percy *et al.* (1991) failed to demonstrate any beneficial effect of naltrexone on the motor or behavioural components typically seen in RS. The study was limited to a naltrexone dose of 1mg/kg/day, and it is possible that a higher dose would have produced different results. One negative aspect of this study is that psychomotor performance on the Bayley scales was significantly worse during the naltrexone phase than during the placebo phase.

In summary, therapeutic efforts with regard to RS have succeeded only in providing symptomatic relief. More specific strategies are hampered by the lack of a biological marker or any firm understanding of the biological basis of RS. Until such time as this understanding is available, prospects for providing more than symptomatic relief must be regarded as limited.

REFERENCES

Nielsen, J.B., Lou, H.C., Andresen, J. (1990) 'Biochemical and clinical effects of tyrosine and tryptophan in the Rett syndrome.' *Brain and Development*, **12**, 143–148.

Percy, A.K., Schultz, R., Glaze, D.G., Skender, M., del Junco, D., Waring, S.C., Zoghbi, H.Y., Jankovic, J.J., Williamson, W.D., Stach, B.S. (1991) 'Trial of the opiate antagonist, naltrexone, in children with Rett syndrome.' *Annals of Neurology*, **30**, 486. *(Abstract.)*

Rett, A. (1992) 'The mystery of Rett syndrome.' *Brain and Development*, **14** (Suppl.), S141–S142.

Zappella, M. (1990) 'A double-blind trial of bromocriptine in the Rett syndrome.' *Brain and Development*, **12**, 148–150.

—— Genazzani, A. (1986) 'Girls with Rett syndrome treated with bromocriptine.' *Wiener klinische Wochenschrift*, **98**, 780. *(Letter.)*

—— —— Facchinetti, F., Hayek, G. (1990) 'Bromocriptine in the Rett syndrome'. *Brain and Development*, **12**, 221–225.

12
CONCLUSION: ASPECTS ON ORIGIN – FUTURE APPROACH

Bengt Hagberg, Maria Anvret, Alan Percy and Jan Wahlström

Rett syndrome is an enigmatic condition. It is peculiar in manifestation, clinical profile and course. It still lacks discriminative laboratory markers for accurate diagnosis and differentiation from other similar conditions. The biological riddle is unsolved, and few hard facts exist to explain its origin (Hagberg *et al.* 1992).

Genetic clues

The genetic basis for RS is now indisputable (see Chapter 10).

- All currently accepted cases of RS are females. This indicates involvement of the X chromosome, even if that does not seem to be the full explanation.
- Twin studies reveal concordance in monozygotic twins and discordance in dizygotic twins.
- A woman with classical RS has given birth to a girl who by the age of 21 months showed a convincing RS phenotype (see Chapter 4).
- Collected data relating to families with more than one RS female support a genetic transmission, working through both maternal and paternal lines.
- Genealogical data from Sweden, going back over seven to ten generations, conform with a genetic inheritance, albeit of quite complex and so far unexplained type (Åkesson *et al.* 1992).
- A significantly increased consanguinity rate, in both maternal and paternal lineages, contributes further support (Åkesson *et al.* 1992).

Clinical clues

As more RS patients are followed into their later years, the disorder is becoming more and more distinct from the group of traditional degenerative brain diseases. Certainly, it represents a progressive neurological condition in the sense of increasing motor impairment; however, the remarkable partial 'come back' in communication, recognition and memory after the end of the regression stage does not fit in with a traditional heredodegenerative disease, nor do the transient advances in gross motor skills of that 'wake up' period which may last for several years. Other arguments are the decreasing intensity in epilepsy in the majority of cases and the development of 'eye pointing' abilities, a compensatory alternative mode of communication, in school age and adolescence. Overall, RS is better viewed as 'a developmental disorder in which the evolving clinical signs are due to the effects of maturation and aging on an abnormal brain rather than to primary degenerative disease' (Kerr 1992). Impaired postnatal dendrite and synapse formation as the underlying mechanism would be quite compatible with the remarkable regression picture (stage II) evolving at age 1 to 3 years, as well as with the partial compensation in later periods of life, when the brains of RS girls might be less susceptible and vulnerable.

Biochemical clues

A statement made in 1988 by Alan K. Percy, speaking at the 5th International Conference on Rett Syndrome in Vienna, still has relevance four years later: 'Only exceptionally in a progressive condition does one see such a relative chemical normality associated with such extensive neurologic impairments.' Huge amounts of non-revealing clinical laboratory data from a large number of patients and deriving from many different centres support this statement. Most likely, the primary cause is not to be found within any of the following groups of neurometabolic conditions: lysosomal storage diseases; lipid, lipoprotein or glycoprotein disturbances; peroxisomal disorders; or purine metabolic defects. Nor is there any tenable evidence supporting enzymatic defects of intermediate metabolic pathways (Burd *et al.* 1990). Studies of urea metabolism by Thomas *et al.* (1990) gave promising results. Dysfunction in nitrogen elimination linked to the urea cycle was suggested. This was further supported by alanine loading tests. However, the postulated carrier characteristics for ornithine transcarbamylase deficiency, thought to be of importance for neurobiological understanding, could not be verified and did not provide a discriminating biological marker.

Another poorly understood deviation in RS relates to biopterin metabolism, of interest due to the deficiencies found in certain atypical hyperphenylalaninaemic mentally retarded children. Zoghbi *et al.* (1989) found CSF biopterin to be elevated in RS patients compared to controls (see Chapter 9). Some years earlier, Sahota *et al.* (1985) had demonstrated normal findings for serum and urine biopterin levels in a series of Swedish RS patients, and a preliminary finding of normal blood dihydropteridine reductase (DHPR). In expanded studies (Leeming *et al.* 1987, Cowburn *et al.* 1988), however, blood DHPR was found to be significantly reduced in RS girls aged 1 to 12 years but not in older subjects. DHPR is linked to a gene on the X chromosome (Armstrong *et al.* 1986). It has therefore been suggested (Blair, personal communication) that in RS there might be an X chromosome deletion causing a reduction in DHPR activity in early life leading to the late infantile mental impairment, which then remains static as DHPR activity returns to normal. DHPR in the brain of one RS girl was found to be normal (Zoghbi *et al.* 1989). Recent Japanese findings of low-normal CSF biopterin levels in a series of RS girls under 5 years of age (Suzuki 1990) do not support a primary defect in biopterin metabolism. Obviously, additional research is needed.

A mitochondrial error of cell energy functions has been mooted (Eeg-Olofsson *et al.* 1990). Changes in muscle mitochondrial shape (Eeg-Olofsson *et al.* 1988), mitochondrial alterations in myelinated axons (Wakai *et al.* 1990) and findings of deviating energy metabolites (Haas and Rice 1985, Burd *et al.* 1990) have been reported. Changes described seem, however, to be inconsistent and vague. Investigations on some patients in the Swedish RS series do not support a *primary* mitochondrial defect (see Chapter 9). That does not exclude the existence of *secondary* and non-specific dysfunction. For progressive neurological diseases, nerve cell death from excitotoxic impairment of mitochondrial oxidative phosphorylation has been hypothesized (Beal 1992). In this context selectively raised CSF glutamate levels in a small series of Swedish RS girls (Hamberger *et al.* 1992) might have relevance.

Very recent studies indicate apparently age-dependent deficiencies in neuronal biosynthesis as a possible explanation. Neurochemical investigations on the brains and CSF of RS subjects by Lekman *et al.* (1991) support an early selective decrease in a specific brain ganglioside, GD1a. This membrane-associated substance is an integral component of synaptogenesis, and is thus of considerable interest in a suspected dysmaturational brain condition. An inborn maturational error could well fit in with the infantile brain growth deceleration and the peculiar stage II regression that characterize RS in the early years. However, these preliminary findings in regard to CSF GD1a could not be persistently found in a larger series (unpublished data). The second finding of the Lekman *et al.* study, a reduction of the axon-affiliated GT1b ganglioside, particularly found in CSF of older RS girls, could indicate disordered axons. Neuronal–axonal manifestations characterize RS females in adulthood up through middle age (Hagberg 1989). Axonal pathology affecting nigrostriatal and spinal pathways ('dying forth' mechanisms?) could also explain some of the motor impairment patterns noted in elderly stage IV RS patients, those with marked rigidity of parkinsonian type.

Infectious and immunological clues
Parents of RS girls often temporally associate the onset of the stage II regression with various common infections, particularly of the upper respiratory or gastrointestinal tracts. A proportion of RS girls also start their regression with dramatic abruptness, and encephalitis has even been initially suspected in some. This suggests the possibility that RS may be due to a slow virus state or a prionopathy of so far unknown type.

Suspicions of a prenatal slow virus infection in a fraction of RS cases were expressed by Riikonen and Meurman (1989). Such findings are of interest in relation to subacute sclerosing panencephalitis-like EEGs developing with age in some Swedish RS cases, as reported by Hagne *et al.* (1989). However, if a slow virus is postulated to have a role in RS, it is hard to explain why it only attacks females. The immunological parameters have been considered in general terms by investigators in Houston, Texas: no abnormalities were found either in the humoral limb of the immune system or in serum immunoglobulin levels in children with RS (Percy, personal communication). Systematic studies of cellular immunity have not been conducted, as far as we know, but there is no clinical evidence to suggest a disorder of cellular immunity. In the Swedish RS series, analysis of CSF immunoglobulins has been performed and no abnormalities were found. Thus, there is at present no supporting evidence for immunological dysfunction in RS.

Neuropathological clues

Neuropathology as well as neuroimaging studies of the brain during life particularly underline the fact that the RS brain is small. That fits with the decelerating brain growth which is a prominent feature in the early years of life of RS girls. Neuropathological examination has not demonstrated any dramatic abnormalities that might be attributed to a primarily degenerative encephalopathic process. Morphological and pathophysiological studies indicate that the major area of involvement in RS is around the basal ganglia. With reduced dopamine and acetylcholine, and degeneration of melanin-containing cells in the substantia nigra pars compacta, this is also clinically evident by the progressive rigidity in later years. Basal ganglia involvement is further substantiated by the reduced number of D_2 dopamine receptors found in PET studies (Naidu *et al.* 1992). Reduced perfusion in the frontal lobes, evidenced by cerebral blood flow studies, and recently by SPECT and PET investigations, should be added (see Chapter 8). Altogether, such pathology could well be interpreted as dysfunction of dopaminergic projections from the basal ganglia and midbrain to the frontal cortex. The recent finding of hypoperfusion also in the midbrain/brainstem area of a 2½-year-old girl with RS (Chapter 8) adds additional support. The early reduced perfusion in these regions might represent not only hypoperfusion but also local nerve cell loss from infancy. That could fit in with the neuroimaging findings of local atrophy on CT and MRI by Suzuki *et al.* (1989) and Nihei and Naitoh (1990). Thus, the immature frontal lobe type hypoperfusion, now repeatedly reported, might be the effect of early infantile deficiencies resulting from cell disappearance in midbrain and brainstem cell structures. The origin of such potential brainstem and midbrain impairment can only be speculated upon.

Future approach

The early infantile and presymptomatic brain growth deceleration, the parallel appearing developmental stagnation, the following late infantile loss of acquired skills, and the general growth retardation through childhood with small trophically impaired 'doll' feet, together raise the suspicion of impaired maturational, biosynthetic and/or trophic cell function. RS brains are primarily miniatures, the suspected silent cell disappearance might be major and the degenerative signs apparently modest. Therefore, transient biosynthetic dysfunction, cell growth or cell life supporter deficiences, or even lack of normal cell death inhibitors, seem to be important target areas to consider for future research. Certainly, traditional growth hormones (Hanefeld, personal communication) and somatomedins (Hagberg 1989) can now be excluded as targets for further biochemical investigation.

Other specific proteins which seem to warrant urgent study are those involved in targets of innervating ganglion cells. Such specific proteins are known to be related to regulation of development and survival of innervating neurons. Continuous stimulation from target substances is necessary for the development and maintenance of normal brain function. Such specific proteins are the epidermal growth factor (EGF), a mitogen for astrocytes, and the nerve growth factor (NGF), necessary for survival and normal development of peripheral sympathetic and sensory neurons originating from the neural crest. Another target-derived protein is the brain-derived neurotrophic factor (BDNF), necessary for the development and survival of specific NGF-responsive neuronal populations. There is also an increasing number of additional yet only incompletely known nerve cell factors which might be of relevance.

The possible arrest in normal development of the neuronal network in RS—a 'neuronal disconnection failure' (Hagberg 1992)—is a tenable hypothesis. The dysfunctioning voluntary movements, particularly of the hands and fingers, added to the findings of Eyre *et al.* (1990) of normal or even 'supernormal' conduction velocity in the corticospinal pathways, provides further evidence that the disorder lies 'upstream' of the outflow from the motor cortex. A 'motor planning' disorder is thus suggested.

Aetiological clues might also be detected from clinical observations besides the more dramatic features of the clinical neurology. One such observation is the surprisingly common infantile intestinal dysfunction (Hagberg and Witt-Engerström 1987). Might an essential gut–brain peptide be deficient? If so, would an approach from gastroenterological research perhaps be rewarding? From very preliminary observations (unpublished) of odd deviations in serine patterns in one of our RS patients, further research on such lines seems tempting. Multi-faceted programmes such as these on previously untouched areas might open new pathways to the final goal of solving the biological mystery of RS.

REFERENCES

Åkesson, H-O., Hagberg, B., Wahlström, J., Witt Engerström, I. (1992) 'Rett syndrome: a search for gene sources.' *American Journal of Medical Genetics*, **42**, 104–110.

Armstrong, R.A., Sahota, A., Blair, J.A., Cohen, B.E. (1986) 'Genetic analysis of partial dihydropteridine reductase deficiency in families with mental retardation.' *Journal of Inherited Metabolic Disease*, **9**, 400–401.

Beal, M.F. (1992) 'Does impairment of energy metabolism result in excitotoxic neuronal death in neurodegenerative diseases?' *Annals of Neurology*, **31**, 119–130.

Burd, L., Kemp, R., Knull, H., Loveless, D. (1990) 'A review of the biochemical pathways studied and the abnormalities reported in the Rett syndrome.' *Brain and Development*, **12**, 444–448.

Cowburn, J.D., Blair, J.A., Mehta, A.V., Hagberg, B., Leeming, R.J., Rutter, M., Surplice, I. (1988) 'Dihydropteridine reductase in mental disorders.' *Biological Chemistry Hoppe-Seyler*, **369**, 527–547.

Eeg-Olofsson, O., Al-Zuhair, A.G.H., Teebi, A.S., Daoud, A.S., Zaki, M., Besisso, M.S., Al-Essa, E.M. (1990) 'Rett syndrome: a mitochondrial disease?' *Journal of Child Neurology*, **5**, 210–214.

Eyre, J.A., Kerr, A.M., Miller, S., O'Sullivan, M.C., Ramesh, V. (1990) 'Neurophysiological observations on corticospinal projections to the upper limb in subjects with Rett syndrome.' *Journal of Neurology, Neurosurgery and Psychiatry*, **53**, 874–879.

Haas, R.H., Rice, M.A. (1985) 'Is Rett syndrome a disorder of carbohydrate metabolism? Hyperpyruvicacidemia and treatment by ketogenic diet.' *Annals of Neurology*, **18**, 418. *(Abstract.)*

Hagberg, B. (1989) 'Rett syndrome: clinical peculiarities, diagnostic approach and possible cause.' *Pediatric Neurology*, **5**, 75–83.

—— (1992) 'The Rett syndrome: an introductory overview 1990.' *Brain and Development*, **14** (Suppl.), S5–S8.

—— Witt-Engerström, I. (1987) 'Rett syndrome: epidemiology and nosology – progress in knowledge 1986 – a conference communication.' *Brain and Development*, **9**, 451–457.

—— Naidu, S., Percy, A.K. (1992) 'Tokyo Symposium on the Rett Syndrome: neurobiological approach—concluding remarks and epilogue.' *Brain and Development*, **14** (Suppl.), S151–S153.

Hagne, I., Witt-Engerström, I., Hagberg, B. (1989) 'EEG development in Rett syndrome. A study of 30 cases.' *Electroencephalography and Clinical Neurophysiology*, **72**, 1–6.

Hamberger, A., Gillberg, C., Palm, A., Hagberg, B. (1992) 'Elevated CSF glutamate in Rett syndrome.' *Neuropediatrics*, **23**, 212–213.

Kerr, A.M. (1992) 'A review of the respiratory disorder in Rett syndrome.' *Brain and Development*, **14** (Suppl.), S43–S45.

Leeming, R.J., Karim, A.R., Sahota, A.S., Blair, J.A., Green, A. (1987) 'La mesure dans les échantillons de sang séché de la dihydroptérine réductase et du taux de bioptérine totale dans les hyperphénylalaninémies et dans d'autres maladies neurologiques.' *Archives Françaises de Pédiatrie*, **44** (Suppl. 1), 649–654.

Lekman, A.Y., Hagberg, B., Svennerholm, L.T. (1991) 'Membrane cerebral lipids in Rett syndrome.' *Pediatric Neurology*, **7**, 186–190.

Naidu, S., Wong, D.F., Kitt, C., Wenk, G., Moser, H.W. (1992) 'Positron emission tomography in the Rett syndrome: clinical, biochemical and pathological correlates.' *Brain and Development*, **14** (Suppl.), S75–S79.

Nihei, K., Naitoh, H. (1990) 'Cranial computed tomographic and magnetic resonance imaging studies on the Rett syndrome.' *Brain and Development*, **12**, 101–105.

Riikonen, R., Meurman, O. (1989) 'Long-term persistence of intrathecal viral antibody responses in postinfectious disease of the central nervous system and in Rett syndrome.' *Neuropediatrics*, **20**, 215–219.

Sahota, A., Leeming, R., Blair, J., Hagberg, B. (1985) 'Tetrahydropterin metabolism in the Rett disease.' *Brain and Development*, **7**, 349–350.

Suzuki, H. (1990) 'Rett syndrome: CSF biopterins.' *No To Hattatsu*, **22**, 609–610. *(Japanese.)*

Thomas, S., Oberholzer, V., Wilson, J., Hjelm, M. (1990) 'The urea cycle in Rett syndrome.' *Brain and Development*, **12**, 93–96.

Wakai, S., Kameda, K., Ishikawa, Y., Miyamoto, S., Nagaoka, M., Okabe, M., Minami, R., Tachi, N. (1990) 'Rett syndrome: findings suggesting axonopathy and mitochondrial abnormalities.' *Pediatric Neurology*, **6**, 339–343.

Zoghbi, H., Milstien, S., Butler, I.J., Smith, E.O'B., Kaufman, S., Glaze, D.G., Percy, A.K. (1989) 'Cerebrospinal fluid biogenic amines and biopterin in Rett syndrome.' *Annals of Neurology*, **25**, 56–60.

INDEX

120